FEMININE BEAUTY

FEMININE BEAUTY

KENNETH CLARK

RIZZOLI
NEW YORK

Contents

To Nolwen

Some time ago Lord Weidenfeld asked me if I would be interested in writing a book on the concept of feminine beauty. I told him that I would be very much interested. I saw from the first that the subject was extremely difficult, and that to treat it fully would mean several volumes. All that I could attempt would be a sort of sketch or introduction to the subject, and even this would have to be limited: for example, I would have to concentrate on beauty as we know it in a Mediterranean and Western European world, and give up all thought of including the concept of beauty in China or in Polynesia. There is a great theme still awaiting someone younger, more learned and more energetic than I am.

I soon found that there are and had always been two kinds of beauty, which I may call classic and characteristic. Classic beauty, which reached its climax in ancient Greece, depends on symmetry, established proportion and regular features. Characteristic beauty treats the features with greater freedom and will allow a *retroussé* nose and small, sparkling eyes, provided that they give the face greater animation. Nevertheless these two kinds of beauty have much in common. Some degree of symmetry is essential, and transitions must be smooth and logical. And then, on the whole, physical beauty must reflect a peaceful or integrated frame of mind. There have been furious beauties and sulky beauties, but they exist in the margin of a calm integrity.

Since, therefore, classic and characteristic beauty have so much in common and so often merge into one another, I have not tried to separate them in the text.

KENNETH CLARK
Saltwood, 1980

The discovery of feminine beauty, like so much that we value in civilized life, was made in Egypt in the second millenium BC. It was a sort of miracle; or perhaps we should say that excavation has not produced a scrap of evidence to explain it. The earliest women in Egyptian art, for example the two goddesses who flank King Mycerinus in a famous group in Cairo (pl. 1), although healthy, well-developed young creatures, cannot be called beautiful. Then suddenly the Egyptian sculptors invented a type of beauty that was not to be equalled until sixth-century Greece. An example of how completely the love of beauty filled the minds of Egyptian artists and, presumably, of their patrons, is the tomb of Ramose (pl. 20). The idea of filling a funeral vault with reliefs and paintings of beautiful men and women is contrary to our notion of death, but it expresses the Egyptian belief that the journey to another world must be made as pleasant as

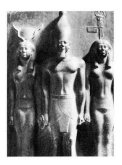

Plate 1

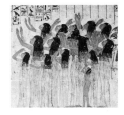

Plate 20

possible. This obsession with beauty reached its zenith in the entourage of Amenhotep IV (Akhnaton), where a sculptor of genius, who seems to have been called Imhotep, portrayed a group of human beings so exquisitely beautiful that we could scarcely have believed in them were it not that the same sculptor did heads of other members of the court which are revelations of spiteful ugliness. Portraits of the Queen who, for convenience, we may call Nefertiti, reveal a delicate beauty which hardly appears again until fourteenth-century France, combined with a sweetness and humanity that we associate with the early Italian Renaissance (pl. 2). Although our present society can have little in common with that of eighteenth-dynasty Egypt, this is still beauty for today.

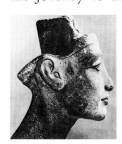

Plate 2

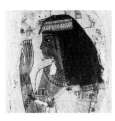

Plate 4

This moment of inspiration barely survived into the period of Tutankhamun, and thereafter Egyptian art relapsed into its thousand years of monotony. But occasionally a relief or a figure of no certain date has survived to show that the delight in feminine beauty had not vanished from Egyptian art (pls 3, 4). Where else could a measure of length be rendered as a beautiful woman with upraised arms (pl. 5)? At some time during this period an unknown sculptor achieved a dazzling piece of feminine beauty, the *Lady with a Wig* in the Cairo Museum (pl. 7). If she was really done in the twelfth dynasty, as the museum

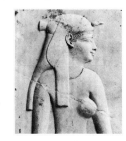

Plate 3

catalogue says, she could be put forward as the first beautiful woman in art.

Meanwhile, the seafaring nations of the Eastern Mediterranean were producing styles as variable and irresponsible as seafront styles usually are. One of these – the art of the island of Crete – achieved, through isolation, a certain character, but precisely what this character was it is difficult to say. The reason for our uncertainty is that the discoverer of Cretan art was the great archeologist Sir Arthur Evans, and the fragments he unearthed were so fascinating that he created in his imagination a whole new style, different both from Egypt and from the almost contemporary (c. 1400 BC) art of Mycenae. Many of the original fragments were completed by a skilful restorer. There seems to be little doubt that when Arthur Evans returned to Oxford his restorer grew bolder and executed whole figures, which Evans accepted with delight. He was particularly pleased

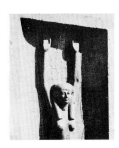

Plate 5

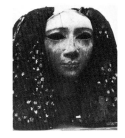

Plate 7

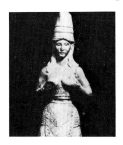

Plate 6

when people said how modern they looked. It is with this reservation that I reproduce one of these figurines (pl. 6). If they are old (which is by no means certain) they support the belief that the beauty of women's faces is dateless. This is confirmed by a unique example of the kind of sculpture that must have been common in the Mediterranean basin towards the end of the sixth century, the so-called *Lady of Elche* (pl. 9), which survived because it had been exported to Spain. A face of classic beauty is encased in a heavily-ornamented head-dress, which was no doubt intended to make her acceptable to a semi-barbarian people of the Western Mediterranean.

In spite of two centuries of scholarship, the origins of Greek art remain profoundly mysterious. What can we say, for example, about that enchanting relief of the birth of Venus known as the *Ludovisi Throne* (pl. 8)? When and where was it

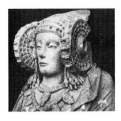

Plate 9

made? What was the original intention behind it? We can only say that here, almost for the first time, we are aware of that gift which Greece bequeathed to European art, an indestructible love of physical beauty. We can study this in a series of standing figures of women, known as the *Kore*. They stood on the Acropolis of Athens, and must surely have had some ritual purpose. When ritual changed and

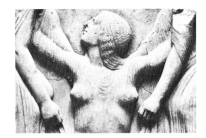

Plate 8

9

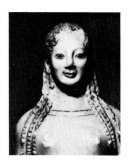
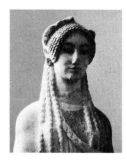
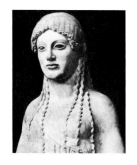
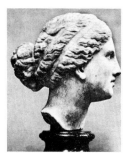

Plate 10   *Plate 11*   *Plate 12*   *Plate 13*

the Acropolis was rebuilt they were thrown away, but have emerged (from the surrounding rubble) remarkably well preserved. The earliest (the so-called *Peplos Kore*) shows the simple column of the body surmounted by a head of adorable vivacity (pl. 10). She is succeeded by a series of almost equally seductive columnar figures, which at first look very much like one another, but when compared more closely (they are all in the same room of the Acropolis Museum) reveal remarkable

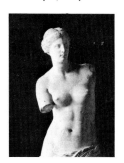

Plate 23

differences both in design and in the character of the heads. Most of them show traces of a gentle smile (pl. 11), but a few are severe and relentless. One of the most famous is curiously self-conscious, as if posing for her portrait (pl. 12). She must have been a famous beauty.

The *Kore* contradict the popular notion that the Greeks were indifferent to feminine beauty, or at least rated it less highly than male. On the contrary, the ideal of feminine beauty that was to have such a long life in Western Europe goes back to Greek art of the fifth century BC, and has remained remarkably constant until the present day. The head in plate 13, which could date from any period of antiquity, is the ideal beauty of the mid-nineteenth century, and would still be taken as an example of perfect beauty by anyone whose taste had not been influenced by the changing standards of the last fifty years. The nose and forehead run in a line which is indented by only a hair's breadth, the upper lip is very short, the ear is far back. All transitions are smooth. The same system is still apparent in what was once the most famous of all antique figures, the *Venus of Milo* (pl. 23), although the head, being subordinate to the whole figure, is more generalized. These heads show practically no trace of human emotion, but by the end of the century the eyes (pl. 15) can look out into an imaginary distance with a certain pathos. A few surviving fragments show that Greek artists had always understood the meaning of pathos. The most familiar remains the most beautiful, the *Mourning Athena* (pl. 14). It is like an

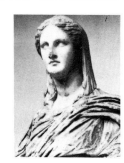

Plate 15

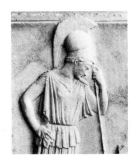
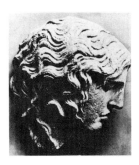
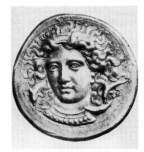
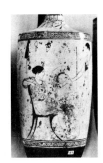

Plate 14   Plate 16   Plate 17   Plate 18

inexhaustible epigram that summarizes a whole complex of thought and feeling. Never again, perhaps, is the female body used with such restraint as the vehicle of deep emotion. One can also discover fragments that show the sentiment which we call romantic (pl. 16), which remind us how incomplete is our traditional notion of classical art.

The classical conception of beauty was diffused throughout the Mediterranean, partly from Greece itself and partly from the colonies of Sicily and southern Italy. The chief means of this dissemination was coinage. Greek and especially Syracusan coins were accepted as works of art, concentrating in their small diameter the finest talents in Hellenistic sculpture. One cannot call the Syracusan decadrachm (pl. 17) a minor work of art; it is a small masterpiece of sculpture.

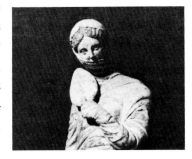

Plate 19

The Greek feeling for physical beauty was also spread by pottery (pl. 18). Just as coins were designed by the finest sculptors, so the leading painters decorated their elegant wine jars with figures which speak to us as directly as a drawing by Picasso. And then there issued from the workshops of sculptors in Athens and Tanagra figurines (pl. 19) nearly all of which represent enchantingly beautiful women. What an aesthetically evolved society they imply! They tell no story, they assert no status; they were simply made to please the eye, and to remind the spectator of something agreeable.

Can we say that Roman art added anything to the concept of feminine beauty? Much of the antique sculpture found in Rome was imported from Greece; we know that shiploads of marble sculptures left the port of Piraeus for Ostia. But it is fair to say that the Roman love of portraiture did produce a few heads of women that add to our concept of beauty, such as a small head of Poppea (pl. 22). They are more individualized than anything that has come down to us from

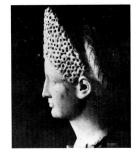

Plate 22

Greece or Magna Graecia. And there are certain pieces of antique sculpture which seem to have a specifically Roman flavour. An example is the *Flora* of the British Museum (pl. 21), a work that, were it not for its impeccable provenance, we should consider an early nineteenth-century imitation of the antique. Anything less Greek, in our sense, than this effusive work it would be hard to imagine.

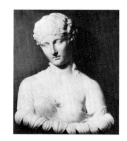

Plate 21

It is always a shock to read in literary sources that the Greeks

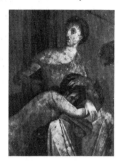

Plate 27

rated their painting more highly than their sculpture, for not a scrap of it remains. But the eruption of Vesuvius in 79 AD has preserved for us a quantity of wall paintings which must, I believe, almost all go back to Hellenistic originals. They tell us that, as we should expect, feminine beauty was more often the subject of painting than of sculpture. To attempt a reconstruction of antique painting on such corrupt evidence would be a mistake. But one series of frescoes, those in the Villa Item (pl. 27), are of high quality, and show us an ideal of feminine beauty of which no precedent in Greek art has survived, although in fact they may well be copies of a lost phase of Hellenistic art. And in the fragments from Pompeii, Stabia and Herculaneum are some very pretty faces to tantalize us with a recognition of our loss. No wonder that the Hellenistic concept of feminine beauty remained embedded in European art long after all other elements of classicism had vanished. Yet this concept was to undergo what seems to us a dramatic change, for no one could apply the word 'pretty' to the ladies who surround the Empress Theodora at Ravenna (pl. 25). When did the change take place? A few surviving works of the late Roman Empire show that it was earlier than we would imagine; or at least that a new type of beauty, which seems to anticipate the style of Ravenna, overlapped with the tradition of classical urbanity. A beautiful

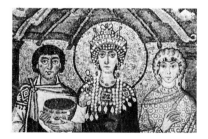

Plate 25

example is an engraved crystal representing a mother and her two children, now in the Museum of Brescia (pl. 26). The oval faces, large eyes, and arched eyebrows are on the other side of that barrier of style which separates Rome from Constantinople. The inscription tells us that it was made in the Greek-speaking East. It could be called the first great Byzantine work of art.

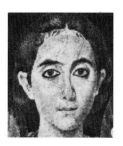

Plate 26

A critic of art in the last century would not have found that Byzantine art had much to contribute to my subject. But today we may feel that a Madonna in the style of Constantinople has a beauty of her own, and it was convincing enough to satisfy the faithful for at least four centuries (pl. 29). But it was more abstract or symbolic than the Greek type, which for some time ran parallel with it. If, today, a beauty in the Greek or Egyptian style were to enter a room, she would be accepted without question; but a Byzantine lady would be isolated, a source of wonder and surprise. As a matter of fact I have known two women (one Italian and one Greek) whose faces required only a slight simplification to become perfectly Byzantine; there is always abundant material in nature to justify any stylistic change.

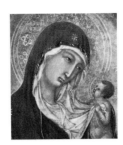

Plate 29

During the disintegration of the Roman Empire in the West, feminine beauty could seldom be the subject of art, for as art revived it was almost exclusively the servant of the new religion. But towards the end of the twelfth century came those first tremors of sensibility that were to produce one of the greatest

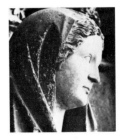

Plate 30

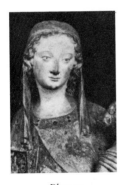

Plate 33

styles in history, the Gothic, and among the many achievements of the Gothic style was a new type of feminine beauty. To a large extent it was based on antiquity. Some of the saints on the north portal at Rheims are genuinely Gothic; others, if their heads are isolated, might well be antique (pl. 30). But in such a figure as the *Virgin and Child* (pl. 33) there is a new rhythm and a new attitude towards humanity, in particular towards feminine beauty. The most beautiful Gothic Virgins are indeed the most refined and exquisite of all types of femininity, and they appear and reappear in European art for almost two hundred years. The *Wilton Diptych* (pl. 28), whatever its precise date, cannot be much earlier than 1400, and it reveals the same ideal of feminine beauty that could have been found in 1200. Not that the later medieval sculptors were incapable of new inventions (pl. 36), and even of an unexpected psychological insight (pls 37, 38). Surely there were many members of the congregation of Notre Dame de Grace who were shocked to

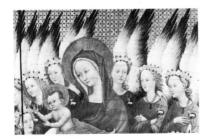

Plate 28

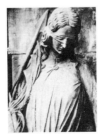

Plate 36

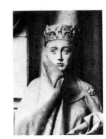

Plate 37

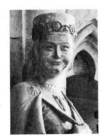

Plate 38

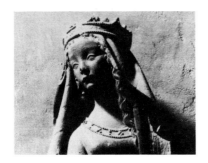

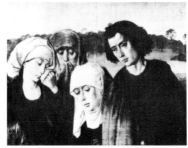

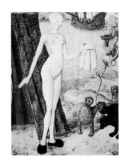

Plate 34   *Plate 40*   *Plate 42*

see Our Lady and the infant Christ turning so emphatically in opposite directions (pl. 34), but they accepted the belief that all images were inspired by God.

In the early fifteenth century the Gothic convention had been compromised at many points. The portrait developed a new intimacy, and in the moving *Entombment* by Dieric Bouts (pl. 40) the painter has made the heads of the holy women into an ascending cry of pain. Women were no longer depicted in virtuous isolation, but as playing a part in a remarkably civilized life. At the end of the century, denuded of their clothes, they appear on a variety of pretexts, chiefly connected with sorcery or witchcraft (pls 42, 43). Thus the nude enters European art, not through sensuality, but through magic and truth. There is a grandiose feeling of truth in Memlinc's *Bathsheba* (pl. 32). On the other hand, Cranach's *Venus* (pl. 41) is an erotic fantasy. He discovered (relatively late in his life) the seductive qualities of a slender body, and created a whole series of elegant Venuses, totally naked except for their enormous hats. These slender, provocative figures were painted in the same decade as the grandiose goddesses of Titian.

The concept of feminine beauty achieved its most complete triumphs in the Italian Renaissance. It may have been more all-pervasive in the eighteenth century but it never reached the same level of greatness. We need think only of Botticelli, Leonardo da Vinci, Raphael, Giorgione and Titian to see in the mind's eye a procession of women, marvellously varied yet united by the seriousness with which their beauty has been portrayed.

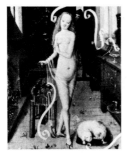

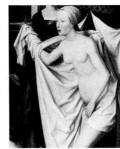

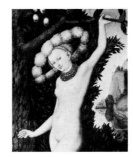

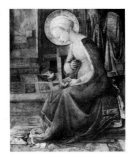

Plate 43   *Plate 32*   *Plate 41*   *Plate 35*

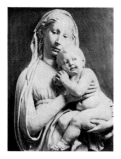

Plate 44

The way was prepared in the first half of the fifteenth century by Fra Filippo Lippi (pl. 35) and Luca della Robbia (pl. 44). Fra Filippo continued the Gothic tradition of idealized sensuality, but made it more individual, so that many of his women seem to us real people whose smiles invite us to form a friendship. Luca della Robbia's Madonnas, although conforming to the imaginative needs of his time, are remarkably truthful. They are beautiful in a rather obvious and undemanding way, so that we hardly think of them as beautiful women at all, but as embodiments of maternal feeling and devotion. Calm, unpretentious, yet often saying the last word in sentiment and design, these Madonnas have influenced our concept of everyday beauty far more than is commonly realized.

Halfway through the century there emerges one of the most fateful of all exponents of feminine beauty, Sandro Botticelli. Since he was first acclaimed by Walter Pater in the 1870s, his Madonnas have filled a place in the average man's imagination previously occupied by the prosperous beauties of Raphael. His early detractors called them sickly, and it is true that very few of them have that look of radiant health that is commonly demanded as a component of physical charm. But there are heads in Botticelli's pictures, like the right hand Grace in the *Primavera* (pl. 57), which seem to me the quintessence of unchanging beauty, and it is hard to imagine a time when they were not recognized as such. They were admired in his own lifetime, and they expressed the mood found in the poems of the leading Medicean poet, Poliziano, the feeling that beauty is delicate and destructible – *per doman non c'è certezza*. The average Florentine wanted something less evanescent, and looked for his ideal of femininity to Ghirlandaio (pl. 46) and Desiderio da Settignano (pl. 45), who convince us that they have portrayed the beauties of their time exactly as they were.

The quattrocento concept of beauty passed out of fashion precisely at the end of the fifteenth century. Its place was taken by an ideal which was to remain in the ascendant for three centuries. This was the creation of Leonardo da Vinci, Raphael

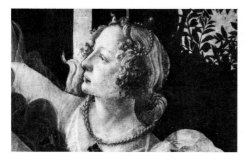

Plate 57

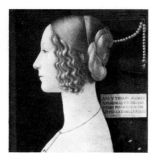

Plate 46

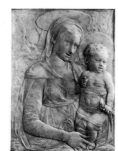

Plate 45

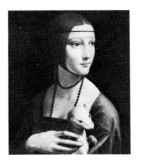

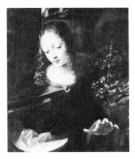

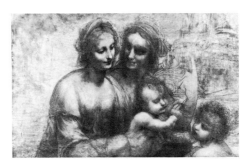

Plate 49   *Plate 50*   *Plate 51*

and Giorgione. Leonardo is the point of transition. His early drawings of women's heads are exquisite pieces of fifteenth-century naturalism, a naturalism which he maintained until the end of the century in such portraits as the *Cecilia Gallerani* (pl. 49). This feeling still shines through the head of the Virgin in the Louvre *Vierge aux Rochers* (pl. 50). Then, in a cartoon for a Virgin and St Anne, he creates the ideal of beauty that is eternally linked with his name. The Virgin is half-smiling, with an

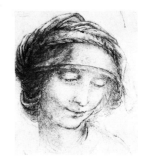

expression which is mysterious but still human – a concept of the Virgin Mary which we may gladly accept (pl. 51). The same expression is transferred to St Anne in a beautiful drawing at Windsor (pl. 52). It is one of the most delicate and mature of all Leonardo's embodiments of feminine beauty. But inevitably it was too subtle for his followers, who continued to exploit the type of beauty known to us in the various replicas of the *Madonna with the Yarn Winder* (pl. 53).

Plate 52

Early in his life Raphael did a painting of the Three Graces (pl. 55) that anticipates in a dozen ways his concept of beauty, both in face and form; but in our present context the key picture is the *Granduca Madonna* (pl. 62), a work of such perfect unity and completeness that one is reluctant to analyze it. It continues the tradition of della Robbia, both in design and in the calm simplicity of the head.

Raphael's mature conception of feminine beauty appears in his great decorations, like the *Stanze* of the Vatican, and he has left us a sort of *pièce justificative* in the

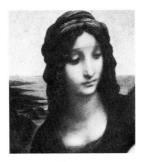

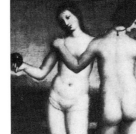

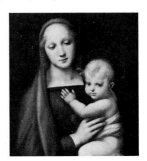

Plate 53   *Plate 55*   *Plate 62*

picture known as the *Donna Velata* (pl. 56), which looks as if it had been done from life, and so may represent his mistress, known as La Fornarina. No doubt it was painted in Rome, under the influence of an antiquity that every day produced fresh wonders. But the round, full modelling is far more naturalistic than the simplified planes of an antique head.

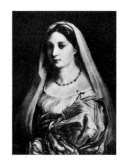

Plate 56

Raphael's concept of feminine beauty had an influence that cannot be overstated. For over three hundred years it was an ideal to which every woman aspired. '*Belle comme une Madone de Raphael*' was a standard expression of praise, and was reflected in the work of dozens of painters from Ingres downwards.

But in precisely the same decade there appeared an alternative concept of feminine beauty – that which was derived from Giorgione and Titian. The *Dresden Venus* (pl. 58), certainly Giorgione's invention although it may have been worked on by Titian, was a discovery almost as conclusive as Raphael's *Granduca Madonna*, and far more influential. (I must record my personal opinion that the head of the *Dresden*

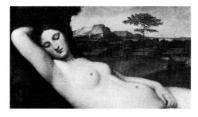

Plate 58

Venus has been much repainted, and may even be entirely the work of a restorer). All the reclining figures in Venetian and north Italian painting go back to this source. The figure has a simplicity that makes other solutions of the problem seem slightly ostentatious. Such perfection could not be repeated, but the Louvre *Concert Champêtre* (pl. 63) is still full of Giorgione's poetry, although some of the actual execution is probably the work of Titian. That the women are nude while the men are clothed shows that Giorgione thought of them as symbols of beauty. He does not intend us to think that this scene actually took place, as Manet does in *Le Déjeuner sur l'Herbe* (pl. 138).

For fifty years Titian devoted himself to the depiction of feminine beauty with undiminished appetite and a wide range of responsiveness, and in the picture known as *Sacred and Profane Love* (pl. 64) he has left us a declaration of his feelings on the subject. There is a glorious naturalness in his response to feminine beauty which

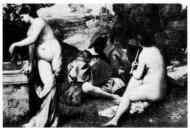

Plate 63

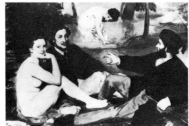

Plate 138

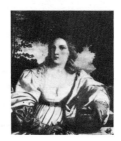

Plate 64

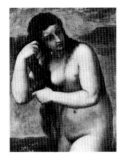
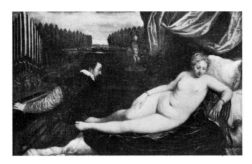
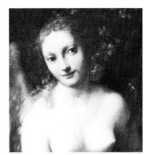

Plate 65   *Plate 60*   *Plate 67*

prevents any thought of mere sensuality, and sometimes, as in the *Venus Rising from the Sea* (pl. 65) his feelings are controlled by an austere sense of sculptural design, so that we do not immediately recognize how unashamedly sensual the figure is. A sense of health and a grateful acceptance of a well-covered body, as in *Venus with the Organist* (pl. 60), lifts our carnal desires out of immediate needs into the happy realm of healthful nature.

Meanwhile a painter of more limited gifts was making femininity his chief source of inspiration; because when all is said about Correggio's contribution to the Baroque style it is as a painter of beautiful women that he will always be remembered. Where did he find these ravishing creatures, whose sweetness and refinement are so different from the solid good looks that we find in the work of his predecessors? They have a self-surrender that has never been depicted elsewhere (pls 67, 68, 69). The answer is, of course, that he found them in his imagination, and the ladies of Parma, who probably looked much the same in 1530 as they do today, made only a slight contribution. His Saints and Virgins make an appeal to us that is unprecedented. They are in ecstasy, and their rapture passes beyond adoration to martyrdom. His *St Flavia* (pl. 70) is the first instance of feminine beauty being used as a means of heightening our distress at an act of cruel violence.

While Correggio was perfecting his ideal of voluptuous prettiness, Michelangelo was following an almost opposite course in a series of heads of women known as the *Teste Divine* (pl. 72). They are amongst the most inexplicable of all his works. They

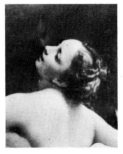
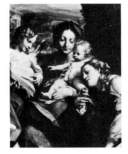
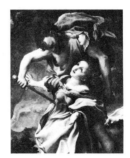
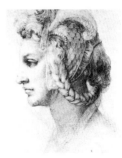

Plate 68   *Plate 69*   *Plate 70*   *Plate 72*

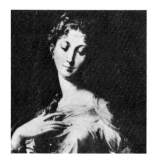 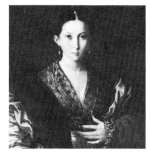 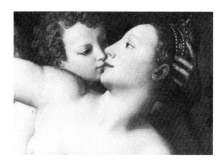

Plate 74   *Plate 75*   *Plate 71*

were probably done as presents for a young nobleman named Gherardo Perini, but why did Michelangelo give them their fantastic head-dresses; why, above all, did he work them up to a condition of finish almost unique in his art? We shall never know. They are a part of his work which is outside our concept of Michelangelo, and are one more reminder of how little we know about him – or about his patrons. We know only that the *Teste Divine* were greatly admired in his own day, and their impassive beauty had an influence far beyond the place and time of their origin.

While Correggio and Michelangelo were at their zenith, and partly as a result of their work, there grew up that alternative to classical perfection known as Mannerism. It was to some extent a negative movement. The great heroes of Renaissance art had gained their ends too completely and left their successors with nothing fresh to say. But in its pursuit of feminine beauty Mannerism was creative, and it introduced the element of strangeness that Bacon had rightly seen as a first condition of beauty. For some reason all Mannerism involves elongation, and never was this defiance of natural proportion carried out with happier effect than in the work of Parmigianino. His *Madonna del Col Lungo* (pl. 74) shows the style perfectly assimilated, and his new concept of feminine beauty is harmonious and consistent. He could extend his ideal to portraiture (pl. 75) without any loss of truth. Mannerism gave artists a better opportunity to exploit feminine beauty than classical perfection had done, as we can see in Bronzino's *Venus* (pl. 71) and the *Diane d'Anet* (pl. 77), whose elegance and latent eroticism make her the perfect *objet d'art* for a civilized court. Indeed in the mid-sixteenth century French and German artists carried Mannerism into a realm of fantasy that it rarely approached in Italy, then in a state of fragmentation, although occasional examples of it there were delightfully extravagant. Many of the results were trivial (pl. 78), or frequently impudent (pl. 79).

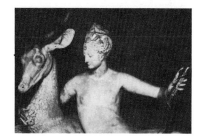

By one of those paradoxes that save the history of art from monotony, the period of Mannerist

Plate 77

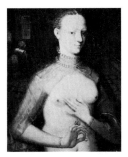
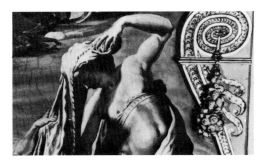
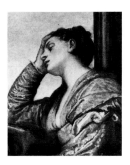

Plate 78   *Plate 79*   *Plate 83*

extravagance also saw the career of the sanest of all great painters, Paolo Veronese. To be in his company for a few days, as is possible in Venice and Vicenza, is to restore one's faith in humanity. His women are beautiful because they are healthy and unselfconscious. We can see that they have never had a mean or malicious thought. It was exactly this unselfconscious candour that was lacking in the earnest and industrious Bolognese painters who, although they almost overlapped in time with the last works of Paolo Veronese, seem to belong to a different world (pls 83, 84, 92). They were the first academics. Before their time it had been assumed that art would simply continue, with slight ups and downs due to the genius of certain individuals. With the Carracci came the notion, which has appeared so often since their time, that art had declined but could be revived by following certain formulae (pl. 81). Academies had existed in the Renaissance only in the sense that eminent artists opened their studios to would-be learners. But from the Carracci onwards an academy was a self-regarding institution with its own dogmas and ambitions. It is not surprising that in such an atmosphere feminine beauty lost its freshness. But among the academic Bolognese was an artist to whom that kind of discipline was unnatural – the painter universally known for two hundred years as 'dear Guido'. His feeling for feminine beauty is present in all his work (pl. 95), but his fame – one may say his popularity – rests on the way he was able to combine this feeling with sincere piety. Rather the same is true of his rival in popular fame, Sassoferrato. He, even more than Guido, had a beautiful simplicity of heart, and his *Madonna* (pl. 82) is

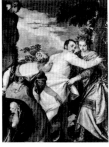
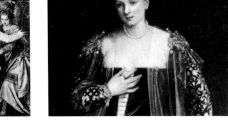
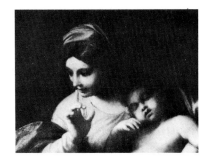

Plate 84   *Plate 92*   *Plate 81*

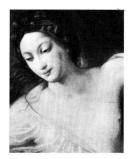
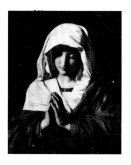
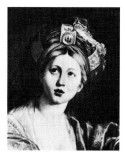
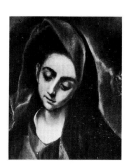

Plate 95　　　　　*Plate 82*　　　　　*Plate 80*　　　　　*Plate 85*

painted with a sort of innocence that will always give pleasure in an uncorrupted society.

The Bolognese artist who gave most thought to the concept of feminine beauty was the serious, industrious Domenichino. As a sideline from his admirable frescoes, he did a series of figures of women which were once amongst the most sought-after pictures of the period (pl. 80). They are designated as sibyls and prophetesses, but their chief function was to perpetuate what he thought most admirable in women. They are not seductive, but quite handsome enough, in an impersonal way, to come into any survey of feminine beauty.

Between the High Renaissance and the great painters of the seventeenth century there emerged one considerable artist who was, in fact, the last and greatest of the Mannerists, El Greco. He was much concerned with feminine beauty; and in his representations of the Virgin and Child (pl. 85) in the Museum of San Vincente in Toledo he creates a type of beauty – a long face, with large eyes, tapering to a tiny chin – which is entirely his own. He also painted one of the most convincing of all portraits of a beautiful woman, that in the Stirling Maxwell collection (pl. 86). But Greco is an isolated figure. No one was aware of his ideal of beauty till late in the nineteenth century. Instead they turned for inspiration to four great artists, who represented the taste of the time – Rubens, Bernini, Rembrandt and Velazquez – who looked at women with new eyes.

Rubens, the oldest of the group by almost twenty years, is the one whose discovery, or creation, of an ideal feminine beauty is most generally remembered, although not always in adequate terms. To the philistine he is simply the painter of fat women, and is thought of as rather a joke. It is true that in his mature work he rejected the convention of classical nudity which had spread from Rome all over Europe, and gave his women the carefree plumpness which, as we know from his two wives, was his own ideal of beauty. But this was always subordinate to a sense of style and a feeling of decorum. In all the vast

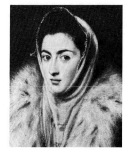

Plate 86

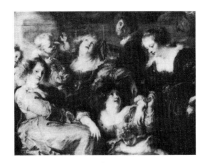

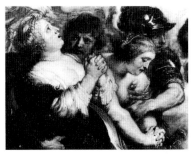

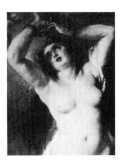

Plate 87 *Plate 96* *Plate 88*

accumulation of naked women in Rubens's pictures there is not one who could be described as indecent. His devotion to feminine beauty led him to invent subjects in which groups of women could be assembled for our delight – *The Garden of Love* (pl. 87) in the Prado is one example, *The Sabine Women* (pl. 96) in the London National Gallery is another – and of course he did many single figures of women in which fleshly beauty controlled by art is the whole theme. The *Andromeda* (pl. 88) in Berlin is a shining example, eclipsing by its brilliance every picture that surrounds it. Yet we must not make the common error of implying that Rubens represented women solely as objects of sensual delight. Such masterpieces as the *Ildefonso Triptych* (pl. 89) contain figures of women as beautiful as any in his pagan fantasies, but devoted and adoring.

The female figures on Bernini's tombs are of the same family as those of Rubens, seeming to be less fleshy simply because they are rendered in marble rather than in paint. They are a joy to the eye. But the finest of his sculptured women goes a little further: *The Blessed Ludovica Albertoni* (pl. 90), whom he has shown swooning in the ecstatic happiness of martyrdom. She is the descendant of Correggio's *St Flavia*, and is equally the work of a sincere believer, which no amount of repetition (and the pose was repeated *ad infinitum*) can cheapen.

Rembrandt's response to feminine beauty is a far more complex question. For one thing he was never seriously influenced by the Italian ideal; and for another his own individual taste affected him so strongly that his ideals of feminine beauty simply

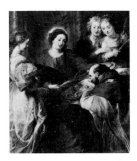

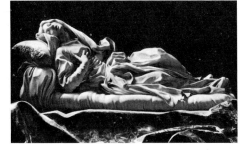

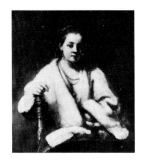

Plate 89 *Plate 90* *Plate 97*

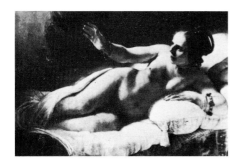

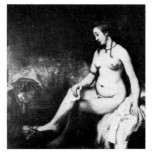

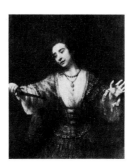

Plate 99   *Plate 98*   *Plate 100*

took the form of the women he loved. We might consider the gap-toothed Saskia as she is usually depicted by her husband – a plain and somewhat commonplace young woman – and Hendrickje's adorable appearance cannot be called beautiful in the conventional sense (pl. 97). The closest Rembrandt came to a statement of his ideal was the *Danae* in the Hermitage (pl. 99), where he certainly wished to make the figure as beautiful as he could. But his love of truth got the better of him. She is sensuous and desirable, but beautiful is not the word that comes to one's mind. And yet when Rembrandt depicts the emotion shining through Bathsheba's face (pl. 98) as she ponders over King David's letter he achieves a kind of beauty which is dependent on inner life and not on physical form. In his last years he painted two women who are beautiful by any standards, both of them representing Lucretia in the act of taking her life; indeed the *Lucretia* in Washington is one of the most appealingly beautiful women in art (pls 100, 101). What led him to treat this subject with such intensity? The Rembrandt mystery deepens at every step.

The missing piece in our survey of feminine beauty is Velazquez. We know that he painted a number of nudes to please his master, but only one of them has survived, the so-called *Rokeby Venus* (pl. 105). It is a work of extraordinary detachment. The model and the pose would normally have inspired feelings of physical desire, but the *Rokeby Venus* arouses no emotions except an admiration for the skill and truthfulness with which it is painted. Can Velazquez have maintained the same detachment in all his nudes? Probably he did, for none of them suggest the kind of engagement that

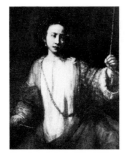

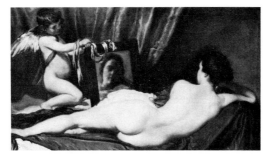

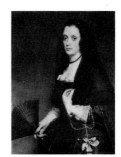

Plate 101   *Plate 105*   *Plate 104*

feminine beauty normally inspires. But he was engaged by the sweet and serious expression of the unknown woman in *The Lady with a Fan* (pl. 104), and has made her one of the most real and lovable women of the seventeenth century.

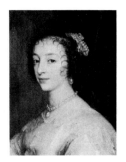

Plate 102

The range of feminine beauty in the early seventeenth century is shown by the fact that almost contemporary with Velazquez's *Rokeby Venus* were Van Dyck's ravishing portraits of Queen Henrietta Maria (pl. 102). They are celebrations of femininity, and no doubt are slightly idealized. Other portraits of Henrietta by Van Dyck show that he knew exactly what she looked like and how far he could go in enhancing her beauty. But the official portraits still give us the feeling of a real person, and we are grateful that he was available to the court when such an enchanting person was Queen. His successor, Sir Peter Lely, was a much less considerable artist, but he too produced a work of sensitive beauty in his portrait of an unknown lady (pl. 103). (Both she and Velazquez's lady with a fan are often referred to as the artists' wives, which may well be true, although there is no evidence for it.)

I did not include Nicholas Poussin in the list I gave earlier because he had a less intense personal involvement with feminine beauty. His embodiments of grace and virtue are suitably aloof, and even his nymphs and maenads do not seem to have aroused in him much physical response. He is more conscious of the meaning of feminine beauty in his religious pictures than in his bacchanals, for example the head of the Madonna in a *Sacra Conversazione* in Edinburgh (pl. 94).

Mythological subjects, which had been so often the setting for feminine beauty, had lost their hold on the pictorial imagination in the last decade of the seventeenth century. But there remained one glorious exception – Giambattista Tiepolo (pl. 106). He is the heir to all the glorious hedonism of the High Renaissance, and he seems, in some moods, to be an uninhibited follower of Paolo Veronese. He is also the last artist to paint on the heroic scale before the arrival of the mighty machine of Neo-Classicism.

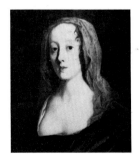

Plate 103

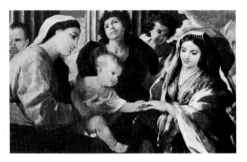

Plate 94

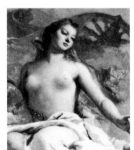

Plate 106

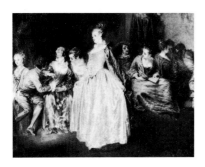

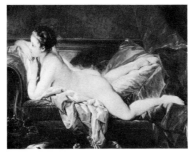

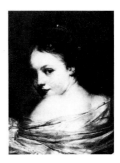

Plate 108   *Plate 121*   *Plate 125*

For the greatest artist of the early eighteenth century was above all the master of a very small scale, who treated feminine beauty with a preciosity that seems perfectly to express its value, and who would seem to be at the very centre of our concept: this was of course Antoine Watteau. He extended our feeling for feminine beauty from the whole figure to the slightest movements – the gesture of a gloved hand or a glance of acquiescence. He used these movements to create a flow of delicate relationships which make our concept of feminine beauty more varied and more

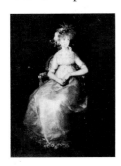

Plate 116

complete. His women come very close to us. They are animated and responsive: we cannot look at them with detachment as we can the sibyls of Poussin. The most enchanting are to be found in his drawings, in which he seems to be telling us about the innumerable possibilities of feminine beauty, discovered in a gesture or the turn of a head, which never reach the point of a worked out picture. Watteau's beauties are rarely seen in isolation. They are usually part of a group of equally beautiful girls, celebrating, by their harmonious gaiety, their consciousness of youth (pl. 108). And yet, as critics have often observed, they are touched with melancholy, as if Watteau could never forget the transience of what he saw. This is what separates him so decisively from his followers, Lancret and Pater, and indeed from other eighteenth-century painters such as Boucher (pl. 121), Fragonard and Greuze (pl. 125), whose preoccupation with feminine beauty was as great as his, but was limited to an enjoyment of its form and its influence on the senses.

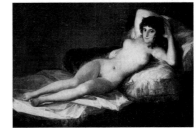

No account of feminine beauty can omit Goya's moving portrait of the Condesa de Chinchon (pl. 116). Instead of the formalized prettiness of the eighteenth century, she has a delicate and slightly disturbing humanity that we think of as belonging to our own time. Goya has also left us in his *Maja Desnuda* (pl. 115) one of the rare instances in which

Plate 115

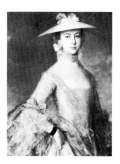

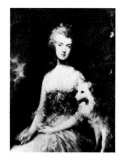

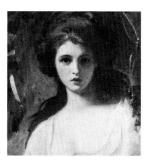

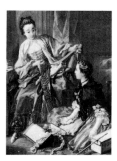

Plate 110   *Plate 112*   *Plate 114*   *Plate 118*

a great artist has recognised the sexual instinct; and yet she is painted so coolly that she awakens no feelings of desire.

In eighteenth-century England feminine beauty took on a more social character. Gainsborough saw it very much as a visible sign of good breeding, one might almost say of good manners (pl. 110), and up to a point he was correct, for a face with all the obvious attributes of beauty, but which lacks entirely the graces of responsiveness, does not, after a first glance, strike us as beautiful.

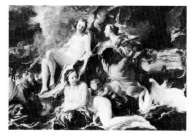

Plate 120

Moreover Gainsborough, being primarily a portrait painter (unlike Fragonard and Greuze), took his point of departure from a likeness, and was much dependent on the appearance of his favourite sitters, like Perdita Robinson. He did not even disguise her squint (pl. 112).

No painter was more dependent on a single sitter than Romney, and we can hardly think of him without seeing in the mind's eye the shadowy likeness of Lady Hamilton (pl. 114). It is arguable that this addiction did him no good as an artist: it certainly limited the very considerable talent that he shows in his self-portrait. But at his best he created an image of feminine beauty which has an almost universal appeal.

I have mentioned Boucher in the context of Watteau, but he must appear again, for his love of feminine beauty overflowed into many subjects. He was a master of genre, depicting his beauties playing with their children or choosing ribbon (pl. 118), and he made them the staffage of large fancy pieces like the *Triumph of Amphitrite* in Stockholm (pl. 120), a banquet of feminine beauty which is almost too much for us to digest.

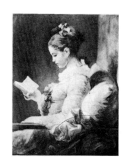

Boucher is a remarkably consistent artist, faithful to his style and his type. In contrast, his brilliant successor Fragonard passes from style to style, from type to type, with a delight which makes him the great wanton of art. But we cannot complain of

Plate 117

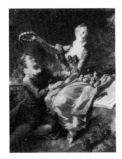

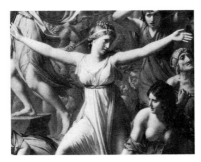

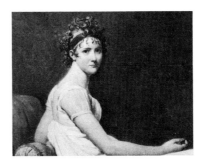

Plate 107   Plate 126   Plate 122

his diversity because at almost every turn he discovers something enchanting, and in the end bridges the gap between the *dixhuitieme* and Neo-Classicism (pls 117, 107).

In the fifty years that are covered by the term Neo-Classicism, say from 1770 to 1820, feminine beauty achieved a position in art greater than at any time since late antiquity. The cult was diffused from France and, in so far as any movement derives from an individual, was initiated by Jacques-Louis David. He thought of himself, quite justifiably, as the master of serious themes, but even in his first considerable piece of historical painting, the *Rape of the Sabines* (pl. 126), the central figure is a ravishing young woman who is using her beauty to separate the rival antagonists. The real subject of the picture is the triumph of feminine beauty. It is therefore appropriate that David is most frequently remembered as the painter of the leading beauty of the time, Madame Recamier (pl. 122). Whether or not the tradition is well founded that Ingres, as David's pupil, worked on the picture, it is certainly the foundation of Ingres's style.

In any survey of feminine beauty Ingres must take a central place. When he was in Rome, from about 1806 to 1812, he was inspired, and in almost every instance women were the source of his inspiration. Some of his greatest images of femininity – for example *La Grande Odalisque* (pl. 124) and *La Source* (pl. 133) – were realized as paintings much later, but we know from drawings that the ideas came to him in his Roman years. They remained at the back of his mind for the fifty years after he had returned to France, and those to which he had not been able to give an independent

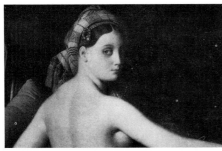

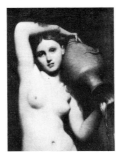

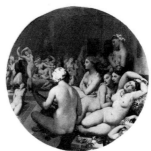

Plate 124   Plate 133   Plate 134

existence were united in that fantastic work *Le Bain Turc* (pl. 134) which he brought to its final form at the age of eighty-three. It is the most densely populated tribute to the obsessive power of feminine beauty in the whole of art.

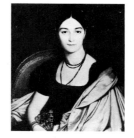

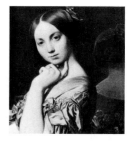

Plate 130

Plate 128

Ingres's admiration of the female form was not confined to these compositions. It was realized, some will think more acceptably, in a series of portraits, of which the most enchanting is *Madame Devauçay* (pl. 130) and the most masterly *Contesse d'Haussonville* (pl. 128). Monsieur Ingres used to say that, compared to Raphael, he was 'so high', bending down till he nearly touched the floor. In front of these two marvellous portraits we may feel that his humble posture was exaggerated.

The Neo-Classical style was the ideal medium for the realization of feminine beauty. Let me give two examples, Prud'hon's *Josephine* (pl. 129) and Canova's *Paolina Borghese* (pl.

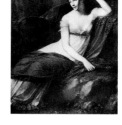

Plate 129

123). They have a grace and humanity that appeals to our own time more than the self-conscious charm of the *dixhuitieme*. We notice that post-revolutionary freedom has been extended to dress. The body is no longer hidden by frills or controlled by corsets, but is displayed in its natural lineaments with pride. That the Emperor's sister should be represented by Canova wearing nothing more than a cast of drapery over her legs was in fact the subject of scandalized comment when the sculpture was first exhibited, but the unquestioned supremacy of the classical convention silenced all criticism. Inevitably there was a widespread reaction, made elaborately clear in Winterhalter's sumptuous picture *The Empress Eugénie Accompanied by her Ladies-in-Waiting* (pl. 131).

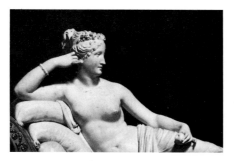

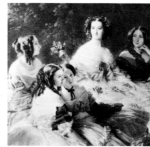

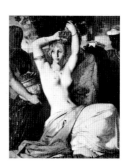

Plate 123

Plate 131

Plate 127

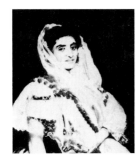
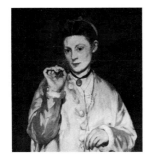
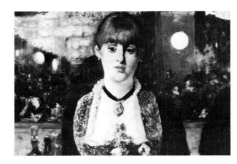

Plate 136   *Plate 132*   *Plate 137*

In the early nineteenth century the nude was felt to have some hierarchic quality. The nudes of Ingres are thought of as goddesses, and one of the worshipful images of the time is Chasseriau's Esther braiding her hair (pl. 127).

The most comprehensive painter of feminine beauty in the nineteenth century was Manet. He saw how differently charm could manifest itself, and his images of femininity ranged from the confident Lola de Valence (pl. 132) to the shy but observant woman with a parrot (pl. 132). His barmaid at the Folies-Bergères (pl. 137) has become one of the quintessential images of the nineteenth century. He also painted the first modern nude, the *Olympia* (pl. 139). What shocked the amateurs of the time was not her naked body – they were accustomed to that in a hundred

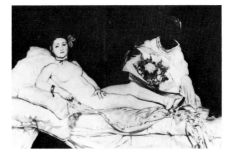

Plate 139

academic exercises, of which Couture's reclining figure is an example (pl. 140) – but her bright, appraising head, which, instead of being a conventional mask, was obviously a truthful portrait. All the same, the number of sexy nudes that seem to have been tolerated in Victorian England is rather surprising. I give as examples a reclining figure by the ultra-respectable Alma-Tadema (pl. 146), and one of many nudes by that tasteless photographer Rejlander (pl. 145). He actually compiled a group of nude figures which was bought by the Prince Consort.

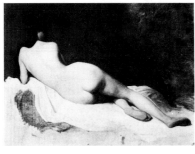
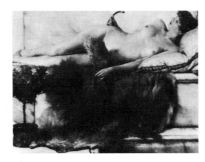
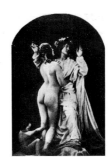

Plate 140   *Plate 146*   *Plate 145*

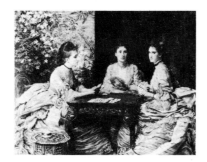
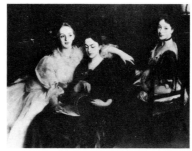
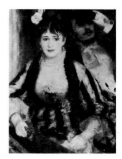

Plate 149   *Plate 150*   *Plate 161*

From about 1850 onwards beautiful women tend to fall into two categories: naturalistic and romantic. For obvious reasons the romantic category is the larger, and this is particularly true of photography, where the essential realism of the medium is a challenge to the photographer's ambitions. A good example of naturalism is Millais's *Hearts are Trumps* (pl. 149), Victorian taste at its most sincere. At least two of the young ladies could be described as beauties, but this is not insisted on in such a way as to effect the unity of the group. Sixty years later Sargent painted a similar group in which the consciousness of beauty is far more evident (pl. 150).

This book shows how the concept of feminine beauty is constantly being given a new inflection. We can all agree about the lady in Renoir's *La Loge* (pl. 161), but might differ over the rosy creatures in his later works (pl. 163). Yet Renoir, who delighted in feminine beauty as much as any man, evidently found them beautiful, and used to paint two or three a day. In our modern concept of beauty, character shows itself more markedly than was once considered acceptable. Virginia Woolf (pl. 169) was not a beauty by any classical standard, but her face reveals an inner life which we value more than conformity to an ideal. An extreme example of how far popular taste has reacted against ideal beauty is Picasso's famous picture *Girl in a Chemise* (pl. 167), which is probably one of the most widely admired images of our time.

But feminine beauty flourishes most naturally in an atmosphere of sentiment and romance. In this genre one of the most wholly committed masters of femininity

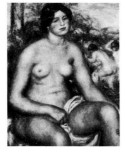
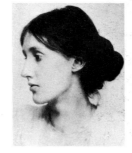
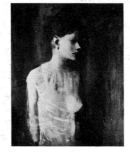
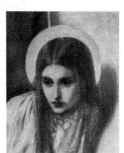

Plate 163   *Plate 169*   *Plate 167*   *Plate 155*

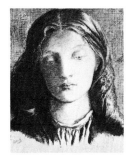

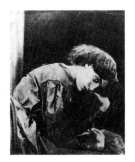

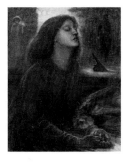

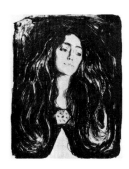

Plate 153   *Plate 154*   *Plate 156*   *Plate 168*

worked in England, although he was very far from being an Englishman – Dante Gabriel Rossetti. An early picture is *The Angel Gabriel Appearing to the Virgin Mary* (pl. 155). The Virgin's head has a poignant beauty which he never surpassed. And this feeling of the face being the mirror of the soul is touchingly present in his drawings of Miss Siddal (pl. 153) and in the picture he painted after her suicide, a tragedy for which he believed himself to be half responsible (pl. 156).

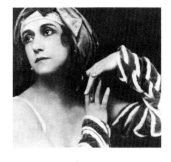

In Rossetti's later work a new and very striking type of beauty appears. This was inspired by an actual woman (pl. 154), the wife of his close friend William Morris. Her relations with Rossetti have remained a mystery, but there is no doubt about his feelings for her, and her marvellous appearance was to influence the concept of beauty for almost half a century. The book

Plate 165

contains other images almost equally romantic, for example Munch's lithograph of Mudocci (pl. 168), or the photograph of the divine Karsavina (pl. 165).

The other English artist to create an ideal of beauty was Burne-Jones. His early work reveals an artist with sharp vision and a personal approach, relics of which are to be seen in the drawing of Perseus and his bride (pl. 147). But all too soon he accepted the taste of the time, and his women fall into a type of conventional beauty that deprives them of vitality. And yet, as we look closely at the faces of the young

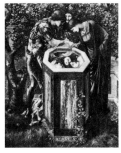

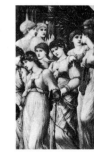

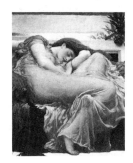

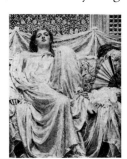

Plate 147   *Plate 148*   *Plate 152*   *Plate 151*

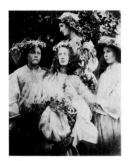
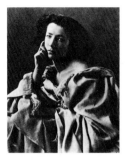
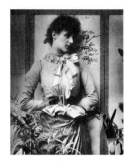
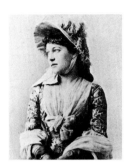

| *Plate 144* | *Plate 157* | *Plate 164* | *Plate 158* |

women descending the Golden Stairs (pl. 148), we see an unexpected variety of beauty for which their highly artificial occupation has not prepared us. This feeling for character in Burne-Jones distinguishes him from his successors, like Leighton (pl. 152) and Albert Moore (pl. 151), where visions of feminine beauty are a vapid reflection of refined taste. From this emptiness we turn gratefully to the camera.

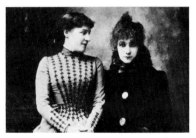

Even Mrs Cameron, all too preoccupied by ideal beauty, cannot exclude a saving element of truth (pl. 144) and Nadar's photograph of Sarah Bernhardt (pl. 157) is more satisfying than the many idealized versions of that famous face. What Academy portrait equalled the photograph of the Marchioness of Granby (pl. 164)?

Plate 159

Of course a synthesis between the ideal and the real is possible, especially when the sitter goes half way to meet it, as in the beautiful likeness of Lily Langtry (pl. 158), and the touching photograph where her Anglo-Saxon solidity is used as a foil to the pathos of Sarah Bernhardt – to my mind one of the most moving photographs in the whole of this book (pl. 159).

We come to our own times, and I cannot say (as one has to say so often) that the standard has declined. Can one discover a type, as one did in preceding periods? Greta Garbo is arguably one of the most beautiful women who have ever lived. Perhaps by rolling into one Tallulah Bankhead, Marlene Dietrich and Greta Garbo

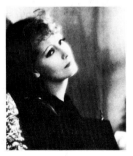
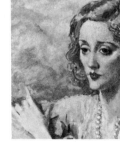
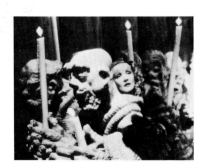

| *Plate 170* | *Plate 160* | *Plate 171* |

(pls 170, 160, 171) one might discover something a little different from any type of feminine beauty that has gone before – a certain withdrawn melancholy and lack of animal spirits. We have all lost self-confidence, and our beauties are not immune. But, as if to show that all such generalizations are nonsense, the book ends with the glorious photograph of Marilyn Monroe on the beach, doing a high kick (pl. 175).

Going back over the plates one has the feeling that, although almost everything else in the world has changed, feminine beauty has remained constant. Praxiteles would have knelt in homage to his countrywoman the Duchess of Kent (pl. 173).

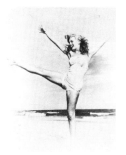
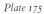
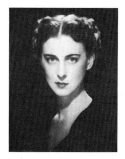

Plate 175   *Plate 173*

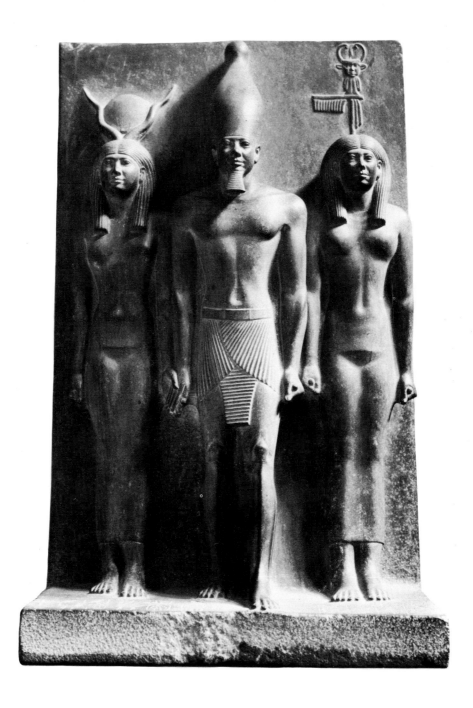

1. ABOVE *King Mycerinus between Hathor and the local deity of Diospolis Parva,* Ancient Egyptian,
fourth dynasty (2590–247 : BC)
Slate (Cairo Museum, Egypt)

This monument, which comes from the temple near the King's pyramid at Giza, is typical of
funerary sculpture of the Memphite Period. The goddesses Hathor and Diospolis Parva, who flank
the King, are executed with their attributes of celestial deity : Hathor, with horns surrounding a
solar disc, represents the sun and fertility while Parva personifies one of the provinces of Egypt. The
presence of the two female figures assures the King's well-being for eternity.

2. OPPOSITE *Head of Queen Nefertiti,* Egyptian, Amarna period (1373–57 BC)
Brown quartzite (Cairo Museum, Egypt)

Nefertiti, who is thought to have married her brother the great Amenhotep IV, was an
acclaimed beauty. Her long, graceful neck and straight profile are characteristics of an ideal
still recognized today. The eyes, under thick painted eyebrows, are strongly accented and elongated
by a painted line : they would have been inlaid with precious stones. There are also the remains of
an elegant head-dress.

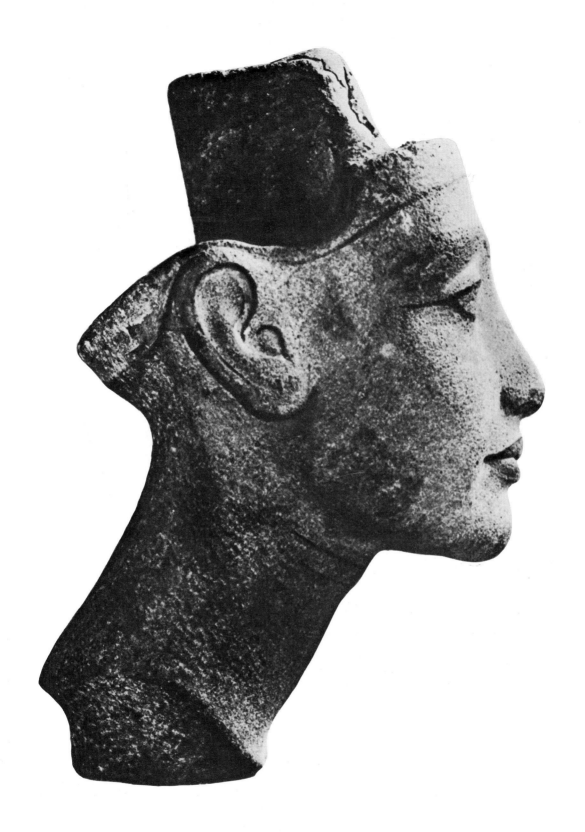

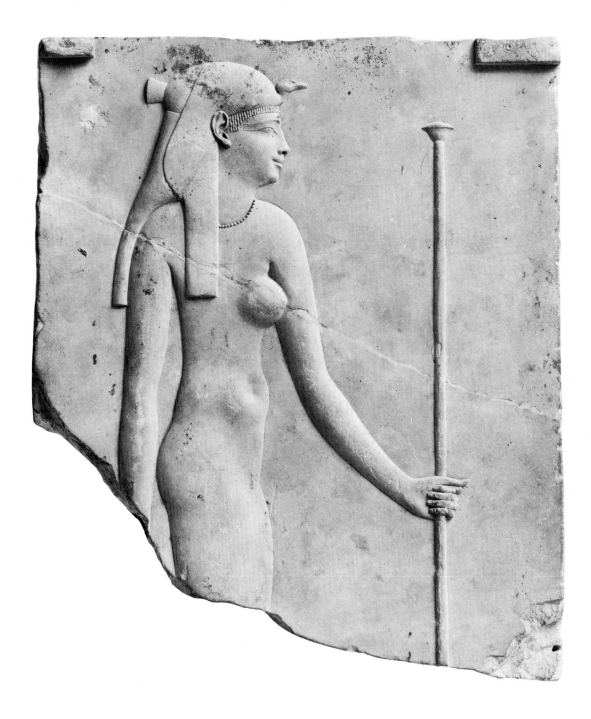

3. ABOVE *Goddess*, Egyptian, twenty-sixth dynasty (664–525 BC)
Limestone (Metropolitan Museum of Art, New York)

This limestone relief of an Egyptian goddess was made as a sculptor's model, and shows the goddess
in profile, naked but for a necklace. Only her tightly curled fringe is visible beneath an elaborate
head-dress. The gentle curve of the stomach and full, rounded bosom indicate a complete
understanding of female anatomy.

4. OPPOSITE *Lady Thepu*, Egyptian, eighteenth dynasty (1567–1320 BC)
Painting on gesso over mud plaster (Brooklyn Museum, New York: Charles Edwin
Wilbour Fund)

Lady Thepu's portrait clearly demonstrates the fact that Egyptians were not interested in realistic
representations of the human figure but in conveying a general impression. They used firm outlines
with flat surfaces, and made no attempt to create a sense of roundness: here the head is placed in full
profile over an almost frontal body. The figure is lavishly adorned with a tiara, necklace and
numerous bangles. A simple gown reveals one breast, and drapery over the left arm shows the
artist's experiment in creating an illusion of transparency.

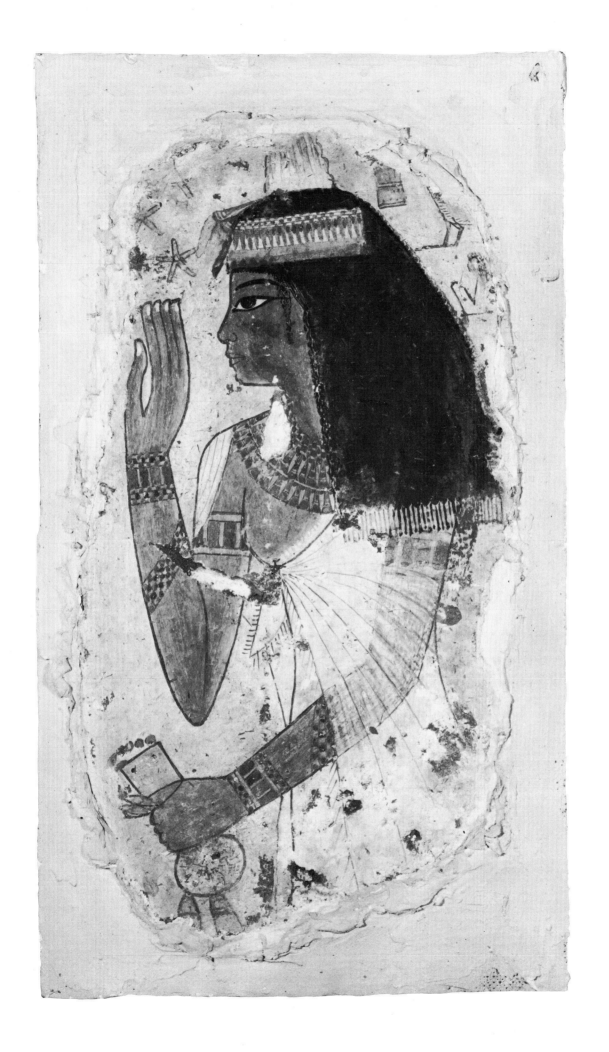

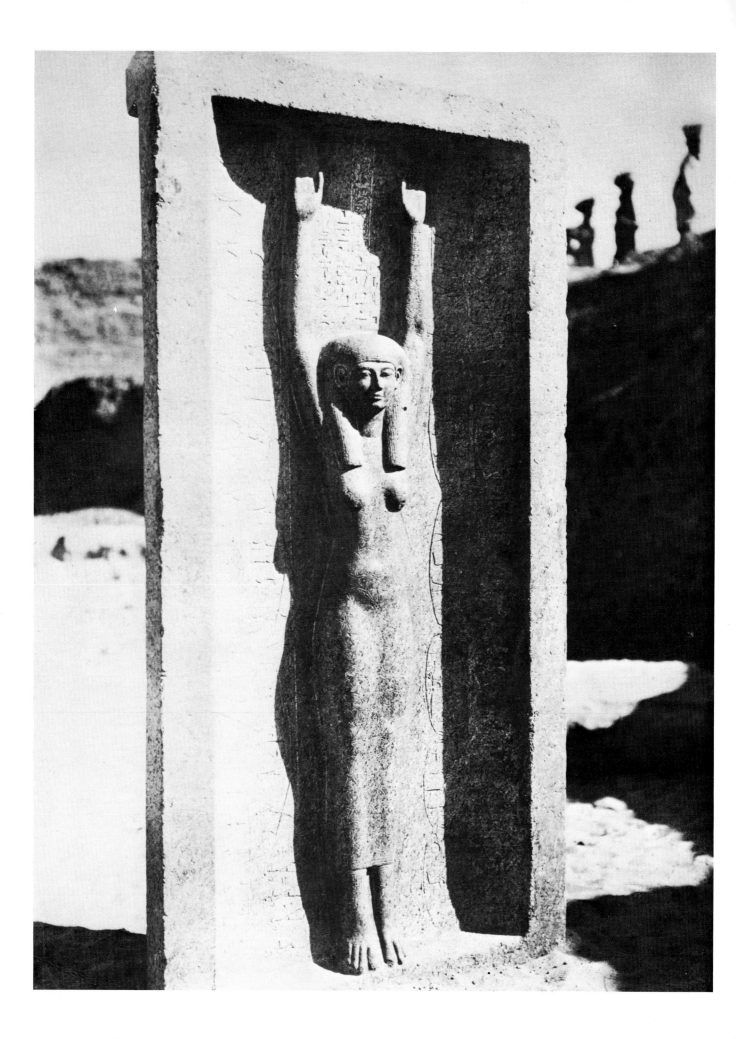

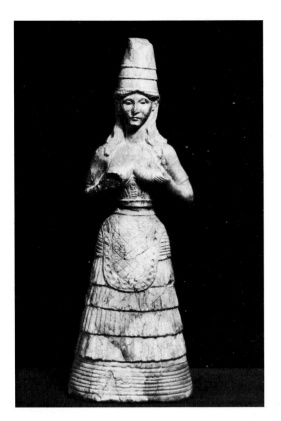

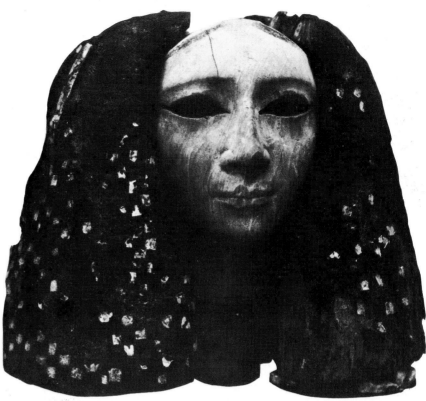

5. OPPOSITE *Sky Goddess Nut*, Egyptian, nineteenth dynasty (1320–1200 BC)
Stone (Tanis, Egypt)

This sarcophagus lid from Tanis is carved with a figure of the sky goddess Nut, to serve as protection to the mummy. It was typical of Egyptian artists to cover all areas with decoration, and behind the figure the lid is covered with motifs and hieroglyphs. The goddess wears a close-fitting shift decorated with stars, which clearly emphasizes the lines of the breasts, stomach and legs. But the focal point of the image is the head, with its large wig, heavy eyebrows, elongated eyes and smiling mouth.

6. ABOVE LEFT *Cretan Figurine*, sixteenth century BC
Terracotta (Fitzwilliam Museum, Cambridge)

This is one of the figurines probably made by Sir Arthur Evans' restorer, and represents his view of Knossan art in the sixteenth century BC. Her elaborate dress, with its tiered skirt, apron and tight waist, leaves the breasts naked in the traditional fashion of the Minoan court. The conical hat she wears is also part of the traditional costume of Crete. The face, however, is 'modern' both in style and sentiment.

7. ABOVE RIGHT *Lady with a Wig*, Egyptian, twelfth dynasty (1991–1786 BC)
Wood with gold decoration (Cairo Museum, Egypt)

Discovered in a tomb near the pyramid of Sesostris I at Lisht, this bust dates from the beginning of the twentieth century BC. The wooden wig, painted black and inlaid with gold decoration, is removable, and it has been suggested that this was in order to change the hairstyle in accordance with the fashion. The eyes would originally have been inlaid with precious stones.

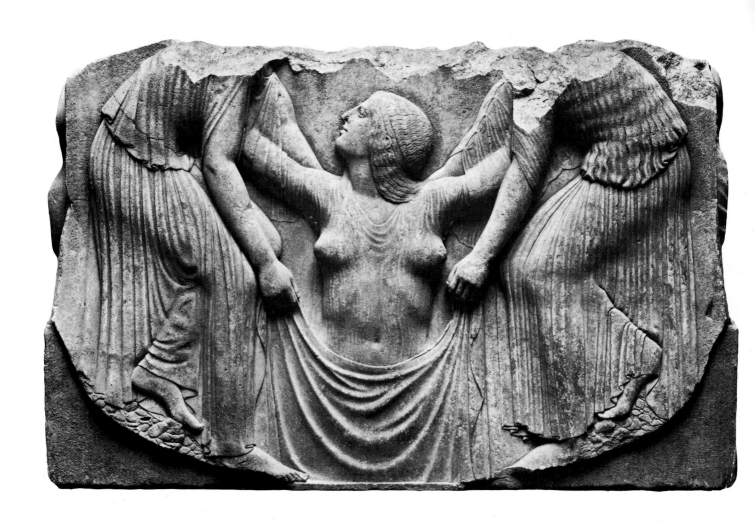

8. ABOVE *Ludovisi Throne*, Ionian, fifth century BC
Marble (Museo Nazionale, Rome)

This marble relief of Aphrodite rising from the sea, assisted by two nymphs, is possibly the front panel of an Ionian altar of the fifth-century BC, discovered in Rome. Venus (Aphrodite), her waved hair held in a fillet, wears a light robe which outlines her shoulders and gives emphasis to the curve of her neck and breasts. This suggestion of sexuality is reiterated in the outlines of the attendants' legs beneath their flimsy dresses.

9. OPPOSITE *Lady of Elche*, Graeco-Phoenician, late sixth century BC
Marble (Prado, Madrid)

Of Graeco-Phoenician origin, this magnificent head was discovered in Spain near a temple of Artemis. The ornate head-dress, with its fantastic decorations and abundance of jewellery, surrounds a face of extreme serenity, and gives a sense of richness which could be understood by the barbarians in Spain. The jewellery is similar to that of statues found in ancient Troy.

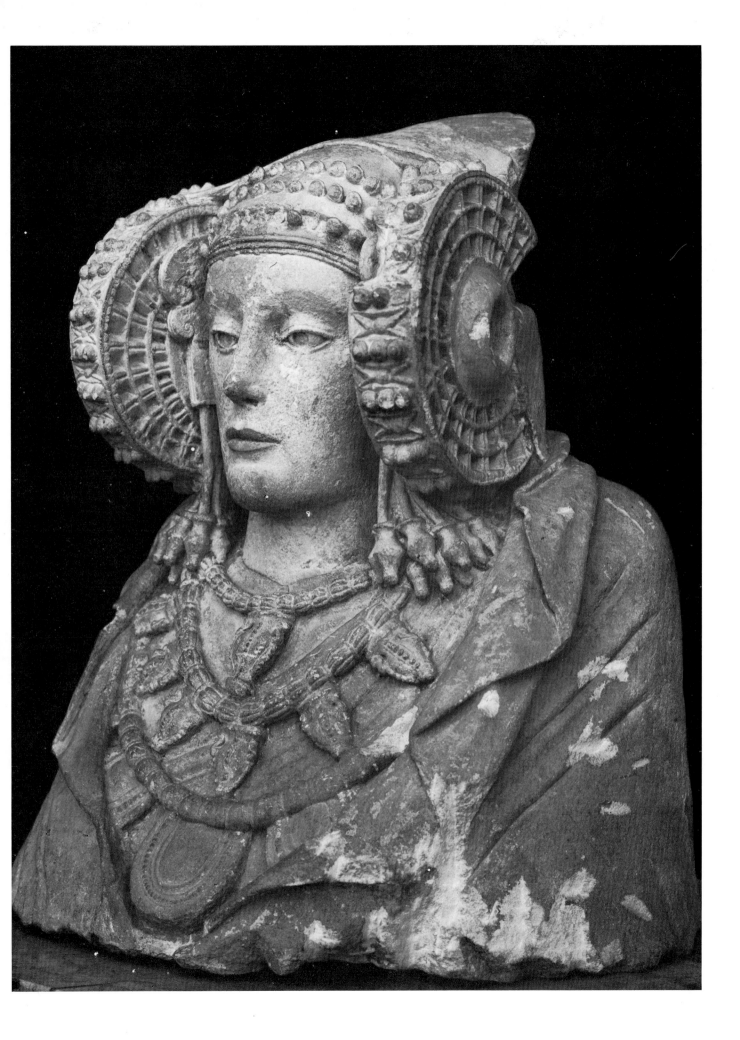

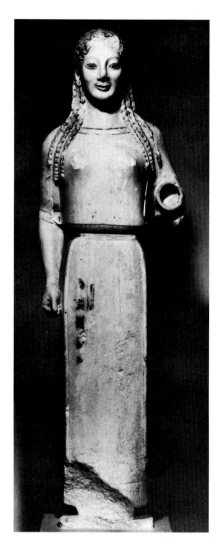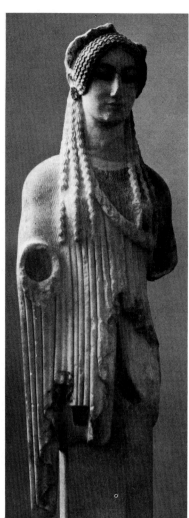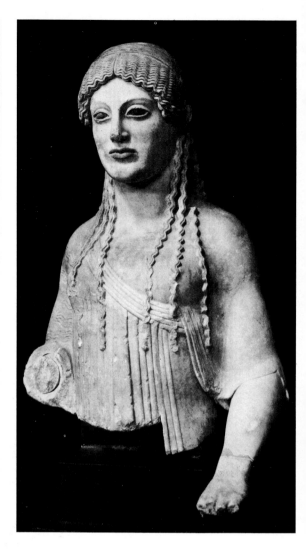

10, 11, 12. ABOVE *Three Kore*, Greek, sixth and fifth century BC
Marble (Acropolis Museum, Athens)

These three columnar figures from the Athenian Acropolis show the evolution of style between
c. 530 BC and *c.* 480 BC. The earliest, the *Peplos Kore*, is charming, but simple and columnar, while
both Plate 11 and Plate 12 show how the artists' style had changed, giving the figure a much softer,
more sensuous appearance. The female figure was rarely portrayed in sculpture during the Archaic
period, but as techniques improved sculptors became fascinated by simulating drapery, creating
heavy folds and diaphanous veils that perfectly complement the female form.

13. OPPOSITE Praxiteles, *Head of Aphrodite*, Greek, *c.* 340 BC
Marble (Staatliche Museum, Berlin)

This life-size portrait, often known as the Kaufman head, is of Phryne, the mistress of the famous
Greek sculptor Praxiteles. She was the model and inspiration for many of his works. Here he
depicts her as Aphrodite, the goddess of love and the embodiment of beauty and sexual attraction.
her hair is swept back in a chignon, accentuating the smooth transition between forehead and nose.

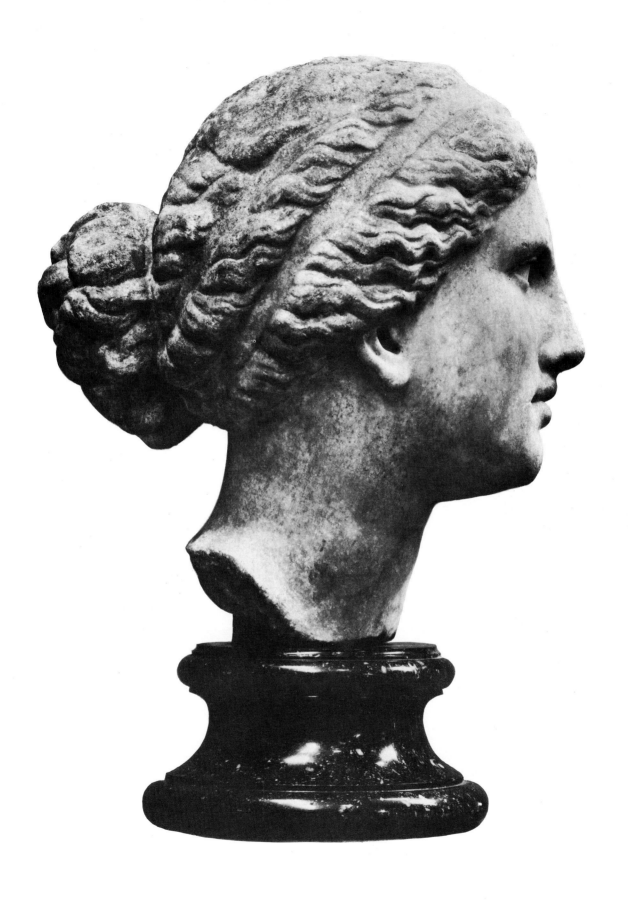

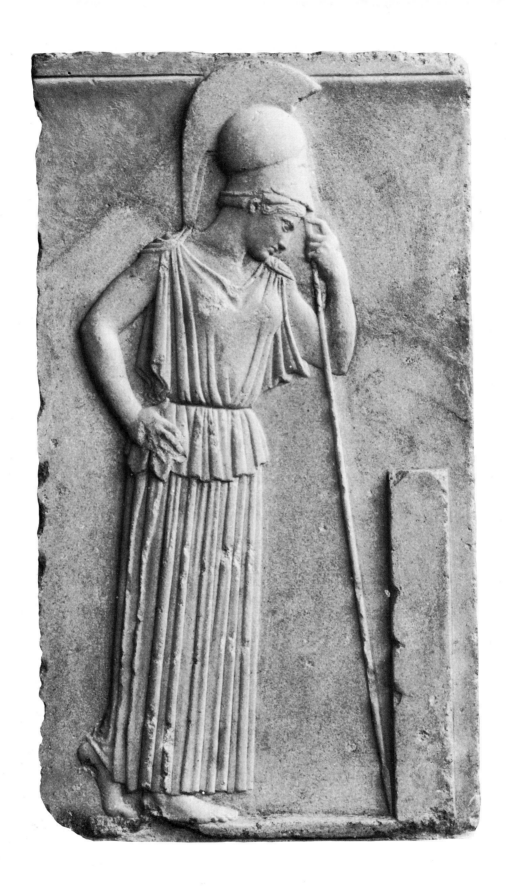

14. *Mourning Athena*, Greek, *c.* 480–450 BC
Marble (Acropolis Museum, Athens)

In this bas relief, Athena, the daughter of Zeus and herself a patron of wars, mourns over the inscribed lists of those killed in battle. She wears her traditional helmet and leans on a lance. Athena is also associated with wisdom, and her downcast eyes and unsmiling mouth give her an air of reflection as well as sorrow.

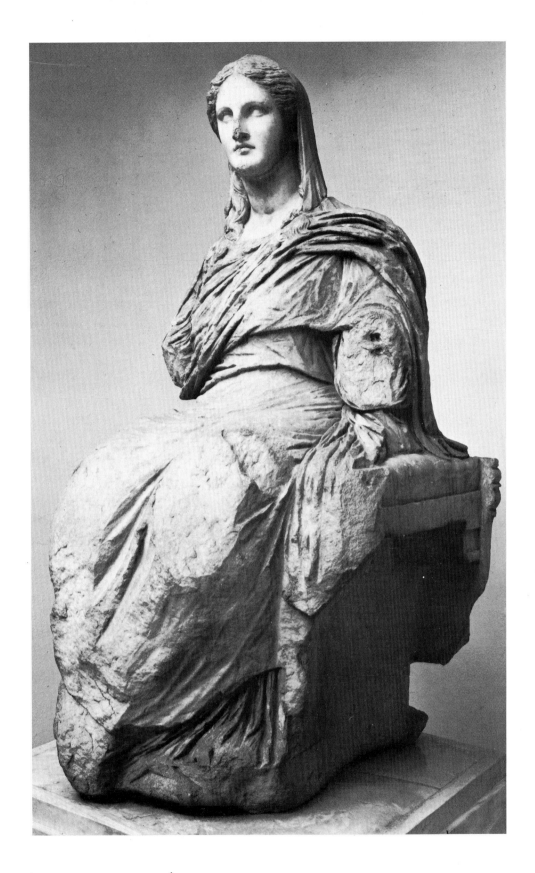

15. *Demeter of Knidos*, Greek, fourth century BC
Marble (British Museum, London)

The earth goddess Demeter's life-size, seated figure was discovered at the sanctuary of Demeter and
Kore at Knidos, and is probably the work of the sculptor Leochares, *c.* 300 BC. The head was carved
separately, in Parian marble of a finer grain than the monumental body, and the serious face with its
deep-set eyes has an intensity of expression which typifies the Phidean's ideal of beauty during the
Hellenistic age.

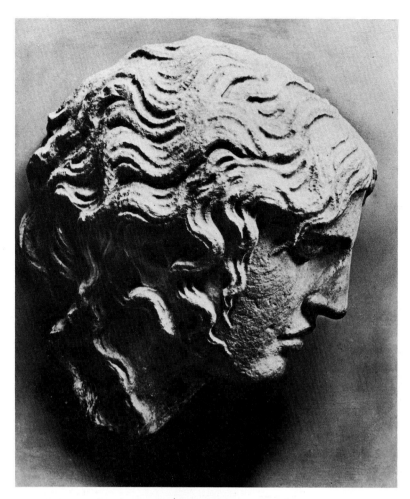

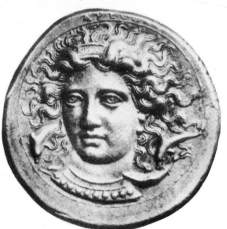

16. TOP *Fury Asleep*, Greek
Marble (Museo dei Thermes, Rome)

In Ancient Greece the Furies were female spirits of justice and vengeance. The Fury depicted here has the straight profile characteristic of Greek art, complemented by unusually wavy, flowing hair. The relaxed mouth, closed eyes and slightly inclined head all create a feeling of gentleness and tranquillity.

17. ABOVE *Decadrachm*, Greek, *c*. 410 BC
Bronze (Private Collection)

During the Hellenistic period the majority of coins minted came from Syracuse rather than Athens. They were often produced to commemorate special events, and here we see an exquisitely carved lady surrounded by leaping dolphins, the attributes of the nymph Arethusa.

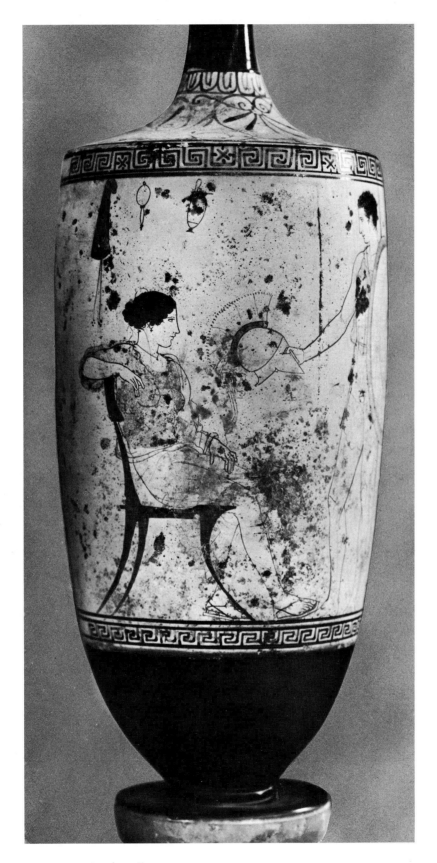

18. *Vase*, Greek Eretia, *c.* 440 BC
Pottery (National Museum, Athens)

Discovered in Eretia, this vase was intended as a grave offering. It depicts an elegant woman bidding
farewell to a soldier. The outline of her body is clearly defined beneath her lightly painted dress; the
delicacy of the work is typical of the major artist of white ground lekythoi known as the
'Achilles Painter'.

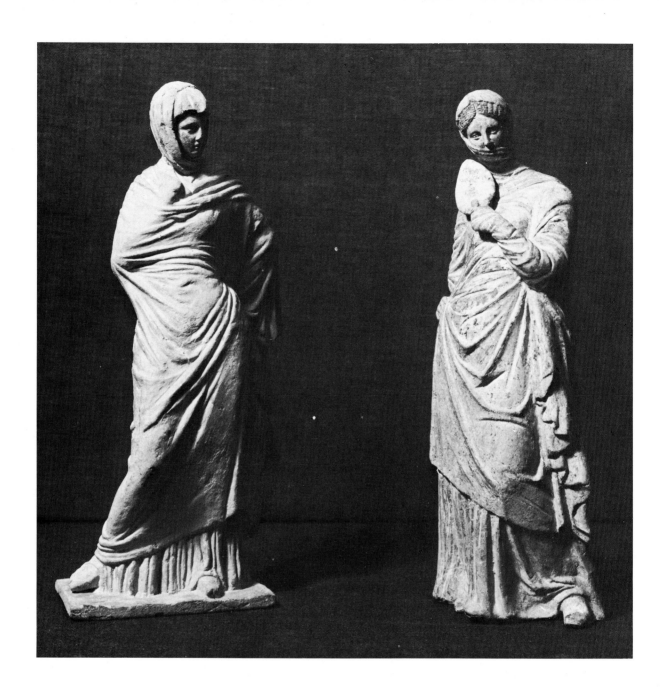

19. ABOVE *Two Tanagrettes*, Greek, third century BC
Terracotta (Louvre, Paris)

Little figurines, about 33 cms in height, were very popular in Greece and widely produced in the third century BC. Examples have been discovered in both Tanagra and Beotia. The costumes, on which there are remains of paint, are carefully draped to emphasize the deliberately mannered poses, and are given an added prettiness with fans, head-dresses and curled hair.

20. OPPOSITE *Scene from the funeral procession of Ramose*, Egyptian, eighteenth dynasty (1567–1320 BC)
Painting on gesso over mud plaster (South wall of Hall of Pillars in Tomb of Ramose, Thebes)

The Egyptians believed wholly in the supernatural and in immortality, and tombs were painted with scenes of human activity to accompany the King to his afterlife. The women depicted here, particularly the central figures, demonstrate the fact that Egyptian artists were uninterested in the backgrounds of their compositions and chose to ignore perspective.

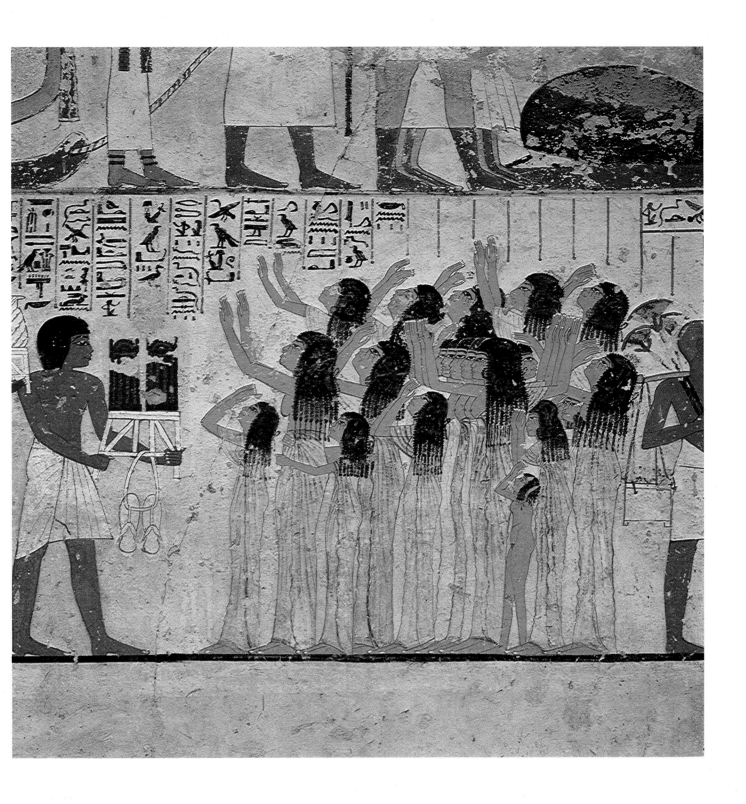

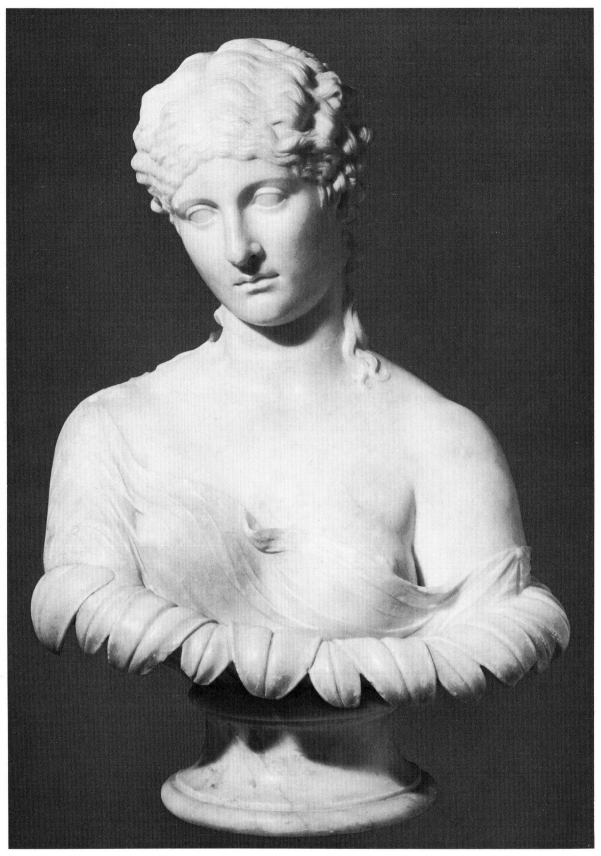

21. *Bust of a Roman Lady*, first century BC
Marble (British Museum, London)

This bust, said to have been found near Naples in the eighteenth century, is probably a portrait of
Antonia (*c.* 36 BC to 38 AD), the daughter of Marcus Antonius and Octavia, and mother of the
Emperor Claudius. Renowned for her beauty and charm, she is portrayed here amid the petals
of a flower.

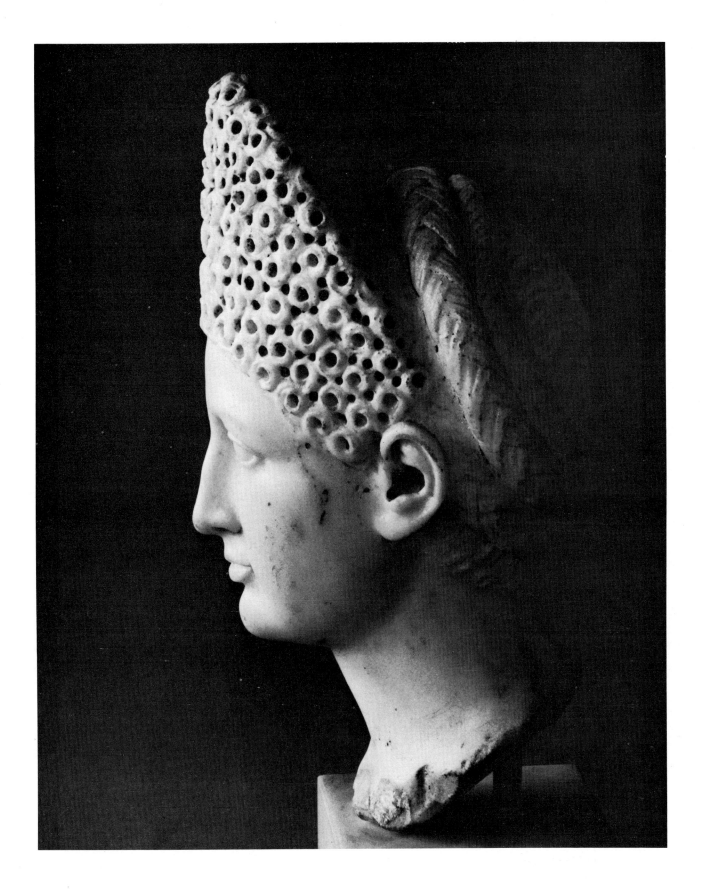

22. ABOVE *Head of the Empress Poppea*, Roman, first century AD
Alabaster (Private Collection, London)

This small alabaster head of Poppea, the Emperor Nero's second wife, is less idealized than Greek portraiture and has a realism typical of Roman art. The highly ornate and elaborate hairstyle, high above the forehead and plaited at the back, was typical of the fashion worn by Roman ladies at the end of the first century AD.

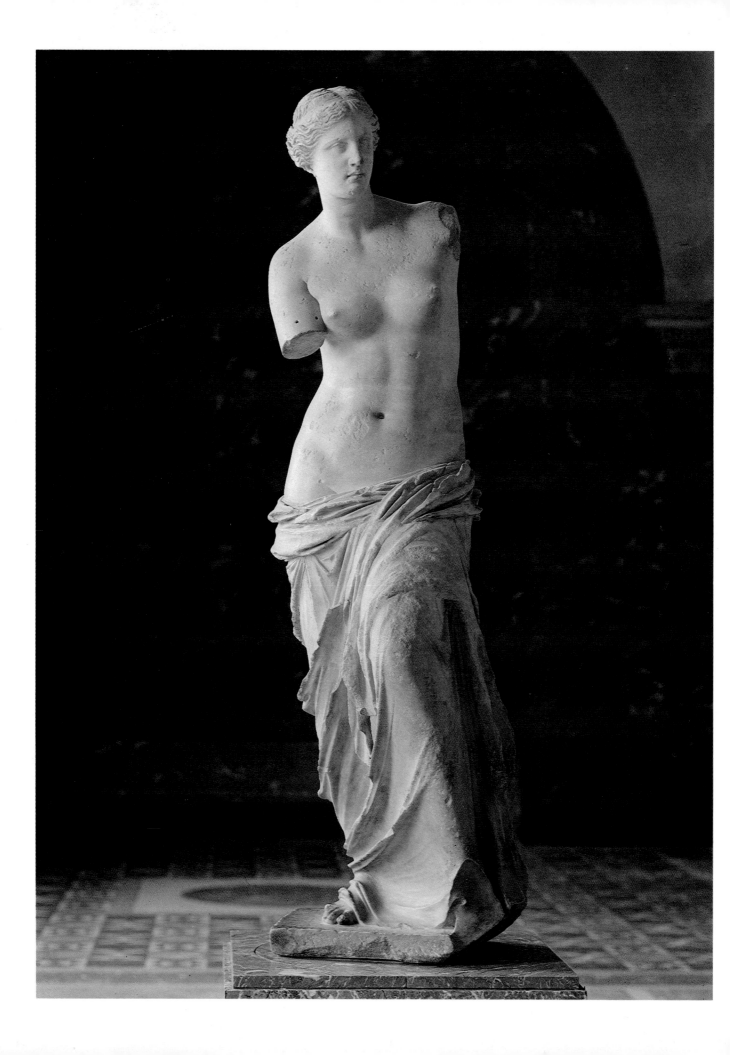

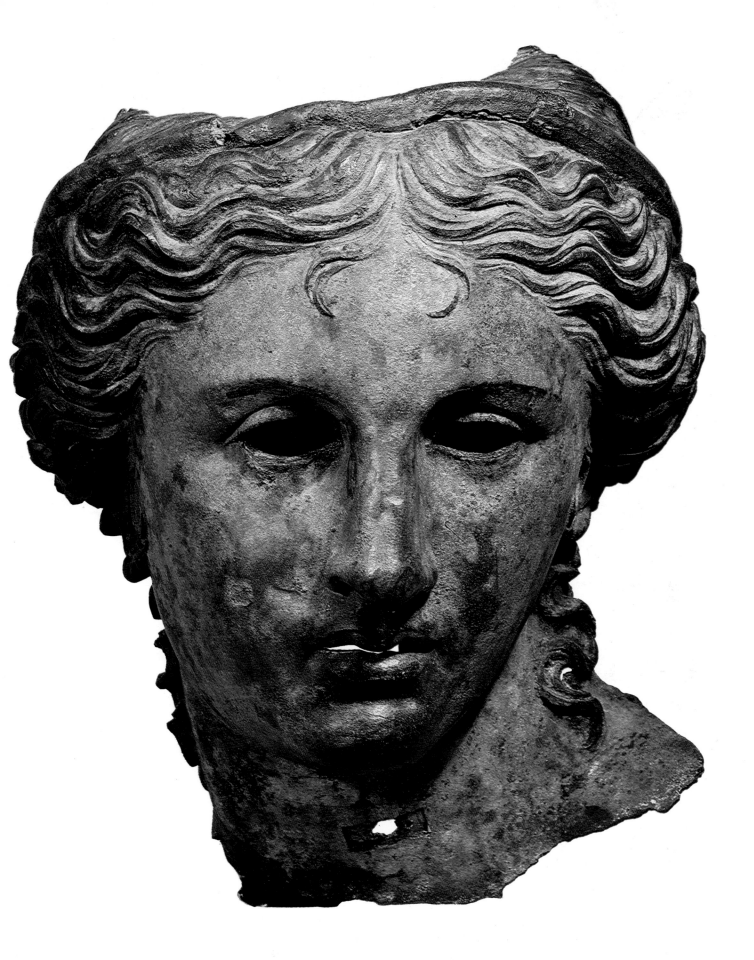

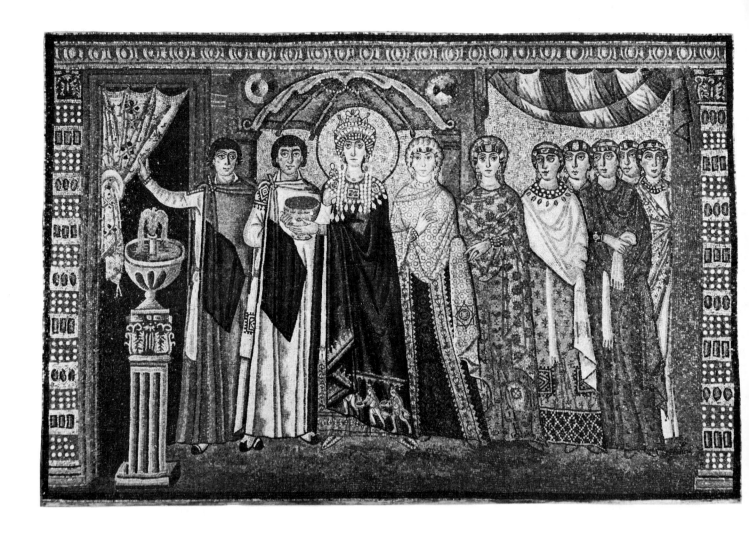

23. PRECEDING PAGES LEFT *Venus de Milo*, Greek, *c.* 100 BC
Marble (Louvre, Paris)

The Venus de Milo was discovered in 1820 on the Greek island of Melos, from which it takes its name. For some time the figure was believed to be a fifth-century original in the style of Praxiteles, but its luxuriant fleshiness and relaxed serpentine composition is typical of the Ionic tradition.

24. PRECEDING PAGES RIGHT *Head of a Goddess*, Greek, second to first century BC
Bronze (British Museum, London)

This magnificent bronze head of the Aphrodite type was found at Sadagh in north-east Turkey. The top of the head has sadly been broken, but the hair would have been worn in a chignon, and tendrils escaping on the neck and over the forehead give a softness to the beautiful, thoughtful face.

25. ABOVE *Empress Theodora*, Byzantine, sixth century AD
Mosaic (San Vitale, Ravenna)

With the rise of Christianity, artists began to portray figures two-dimensionally, reducing forms to an icon-like flat frontality. An example is this magnificent Byzantine mosaic of the Emperor Justinian's wife, Theodora. Her heavily painted eyebrows, accentuated eyes and elongated features are all effects of the eastern influence resulting from the union of east and west under Constantine in 311 AD. The mosaic has been much restored.

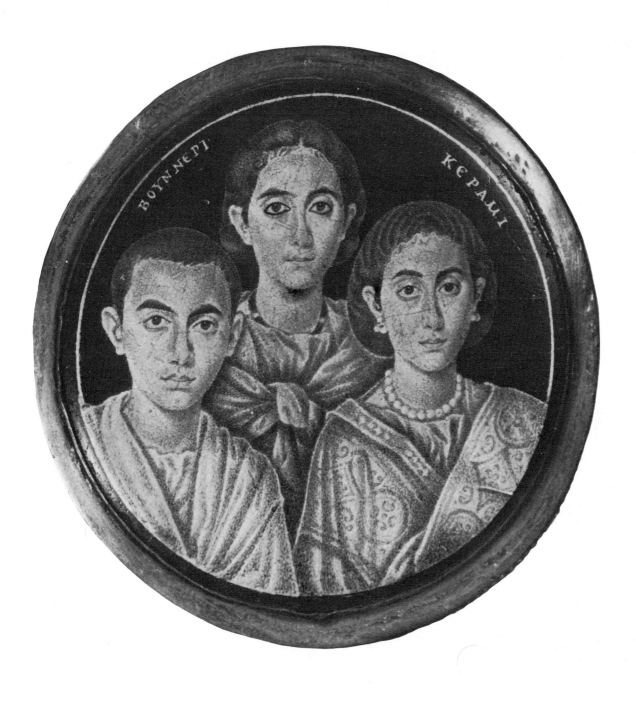

26. ABOVE *Galla Placidia and Her Children*, Graeco-Roman, *c.* 430 AD
Gold leaf on glass (Brescia Museum)

This is the only surviving icon of the famous Empress Galla Placidia, the daughter of Theodosus, who ruled the western world. The distinctly different faces of the Empress (centre) and her children show the extent to which individualism had entered the art of portraiture. Galla Placidia's large eyes, heavily outlined, convey her strength of character. This exquisite glass roundel is set into a gold cross.

27. OVERLEAF *Group of women*, Roman, first century AD
Fresco (Villa Item, Pompeii)

This fresco is one of a series, illustrating the story of Bacchus and Ariadne, in the Villa Item near Pompeii, also known as the Villa of the Mysteries. Depicting one of the initiation rites of Bacchus, it shows a girl protecting herself from a winged demon (who appears on another wall of the room) as he prepares to whip her. In the foreground is a dancing nude Bacchant.

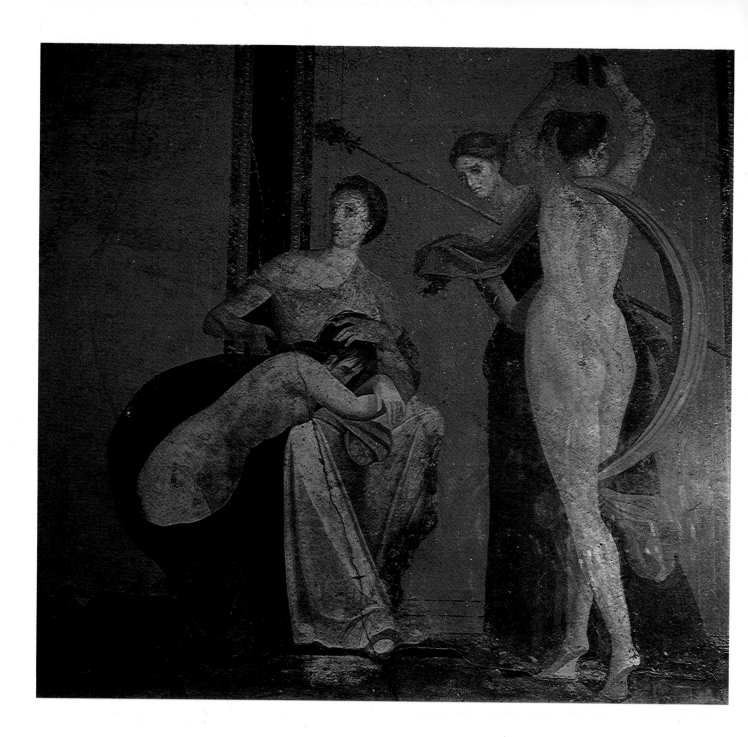

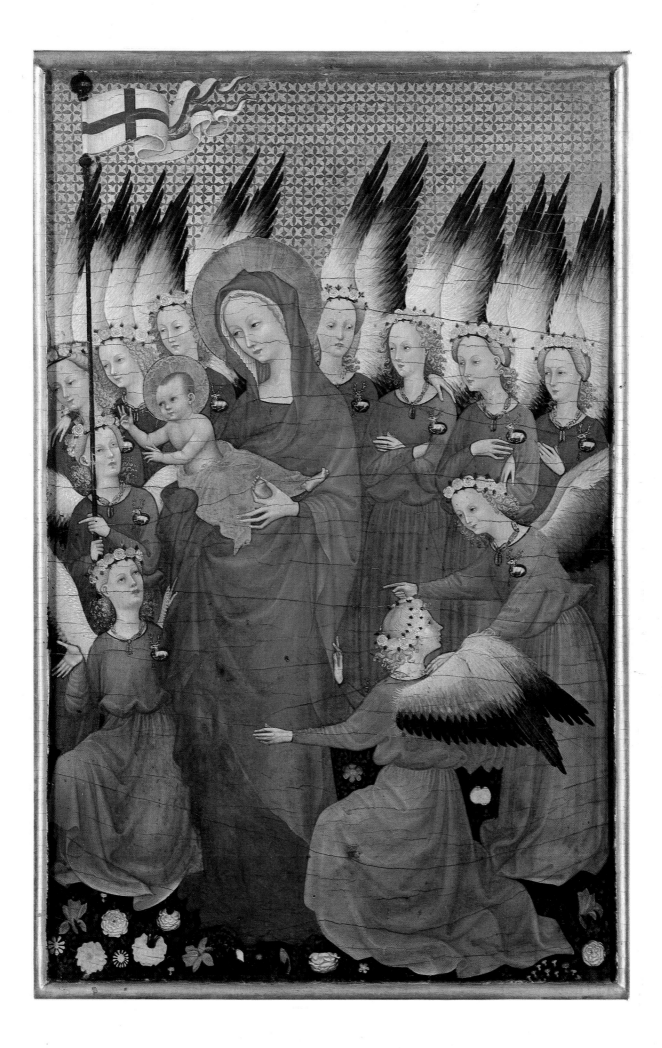

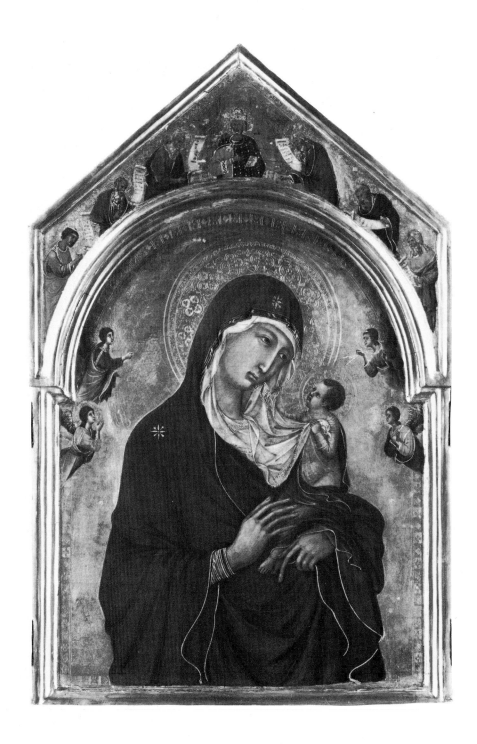

28. PRECEDING PAGE French School, *Wilton Diptych* (right panel), *c.* 1395 or later
Wood (National Gallery, London)

Colour and movement combine in this testament to Gothic feminine beauty. The Virgin and Child, with their host of angels, smile benignly on the kneeling Richard II and saints, who occupy the opposite panel. The angels wear on their tunics the white hart and peascod collar, which were the King's personal emblems. Their small, stylized faces are framed by garlands of roses.

29. ABOVE Duccio di Buoninsegna, *The Virgin and Child* (centre panel of a triptych), probably before 1318
Wood (National Gallery, London)

The stylized lines of the Madonna's face echo a tradition which stretches back centuries: she is still the essence of formal, austere Byzantine beauty, but a subtlety of colour and movement transform her, heralding the approach of a new humanity.

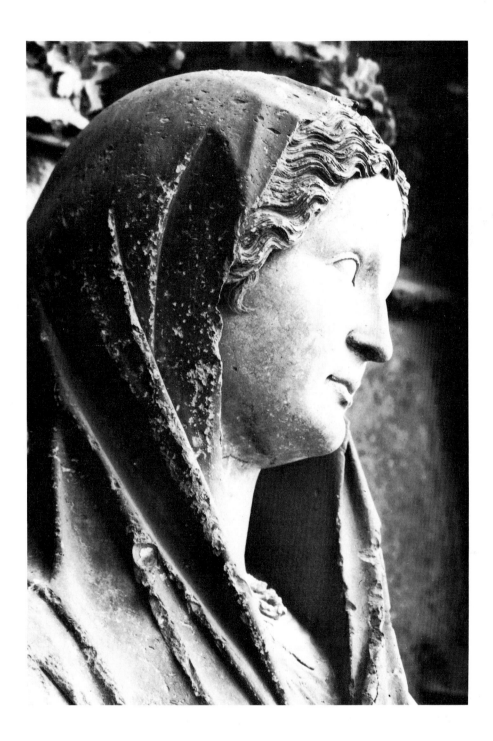

30. ABOVE *The Virgin of the Visitation* (detail), *c.* 1225–45
Stone (Central door of Rheims Cathedral)

This figure of the Virgin, which decorates the jamb of the central door at Rheims Cathedral, forms part of a group enacting the narrative of the Visitation. The rather solid face and figure are reminiscent of a Roman matron, and her physical features and mode of dress must surely have been inspired by Roman sculpture.

31. OVERLEAF Martin Schongauer, *Madonna of the Rose Bower*, 1473
Wood (St Martin's, Colmar)

This is the only painting definitely attributable to the German painter and engraver Schongauer, who was influenced by Rogier van der Weyden and other Netherlandish artists, and whose famous series of 115 engravings had an important influence on German art in general and on Dürer in particular. Jewel-like colours and highly decorative attention to detail give the impression of its being a small painting, but the figure of the Madonna is in fact over life size.

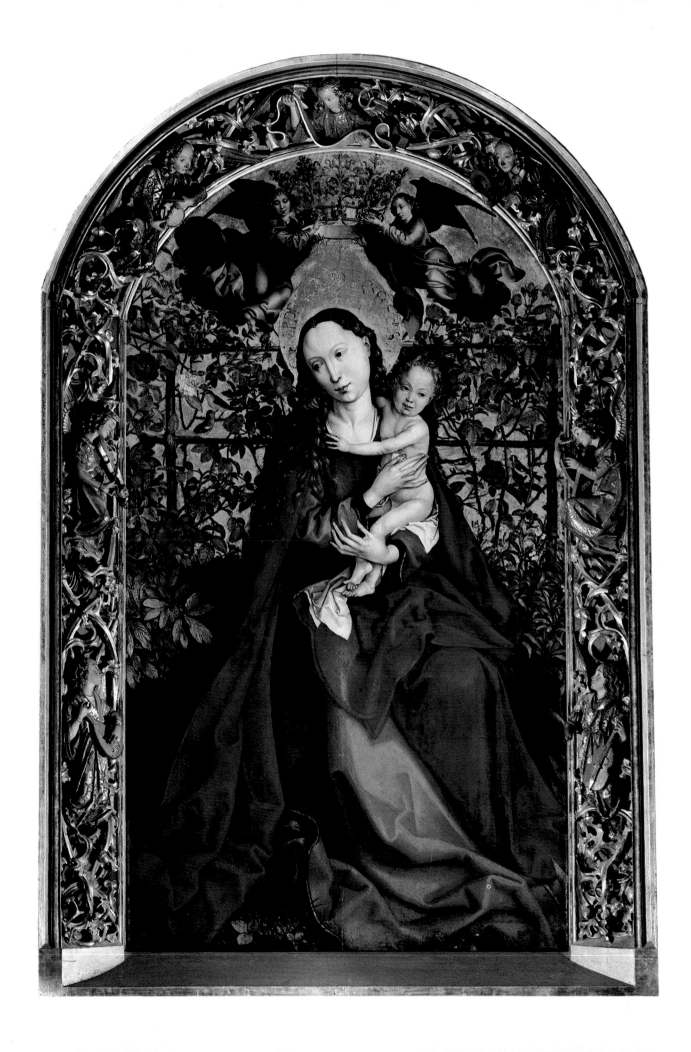

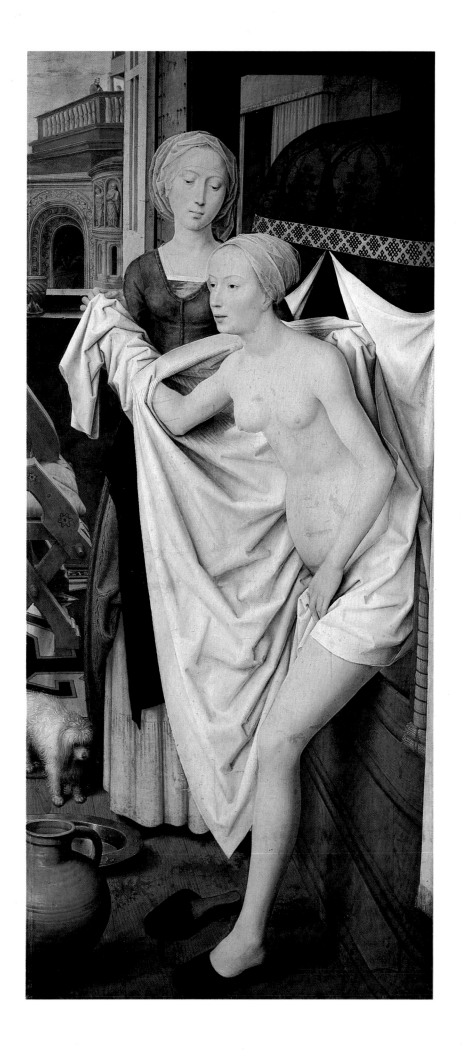

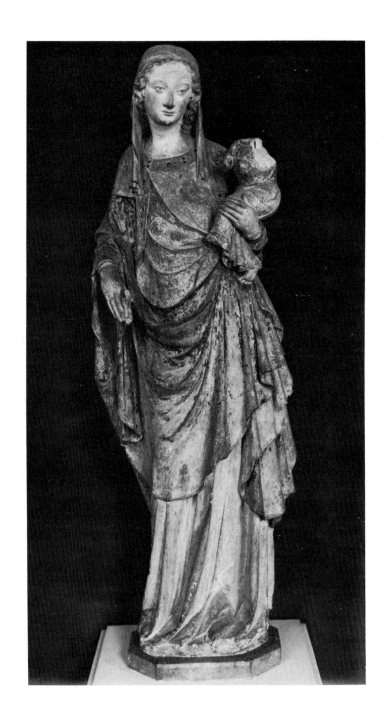

32. PRECEDING PAGE Hans Memlinc, *Bathsheba*
Wood (Staatsgalerie, Stuttgart)

The slender body of Bathsheba is in an alternative convention to the classical law of proportion: her distended stomach and high breasts are hallmarks of the Netherlandish nudes of the period. This strange shape derives from the Gothic attitude to nakedness and a shame of the female form, and not, as in Italy, from the classical ideal. Memlinc's Bathsheba, however, has a monumentality and honesty that belies her origins.

33. ABOVE *Virgin and Child*, first quarter of the fourteenth-century
Painted stone (Louvre, Paris)

Discovered in the church tower at La Celle, near Paris, this free-standing sculpture was acquired by the Louvre in 1905. It had been coated in modern paint, but restoration revealed a delicate original colour – enhanced by inset precious stones – and a face of immense charm and tenderness. The Virgin's regular features make her a perfect example of the refined work being done by Parisian sculptors at the time, a reaction against the monumental style of the late thirteenth-century.

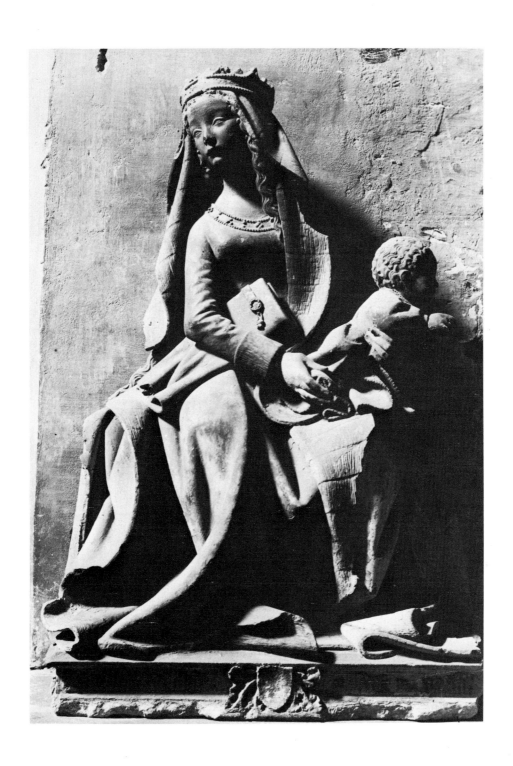

34. *Virgin and Child*
Stone (Notre Dame de Grace, Toulouse)

This statue of the Virgin and Child in Toulouse Cathedral is quite different in character from the formal representation of the 'Madonna Enthroned' of the early Gothic period. Her small, pretty face and natural pose must have shocked those who were not accustomed to such individual portrayals of the Holy Virgin.

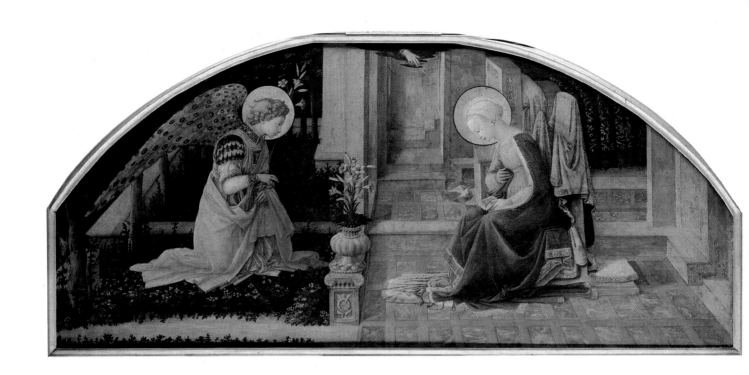

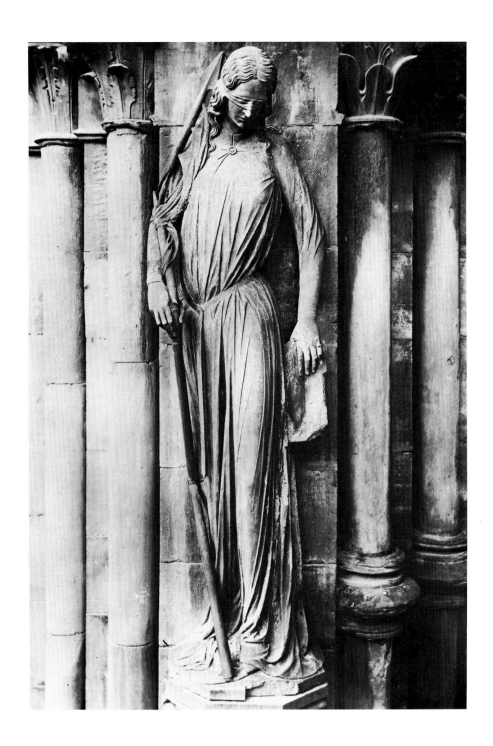

35. OPPOSITE Fra Filippo Lippi, *The Annunciation, c.* 1448
Wood (National Gallery, London)

The Medici family were patrons to Lippi at the time he painted *The Annunciation*, which was destined as an overdoor panel in the Palazzo Medici. The scene could well have been set in the courtyard of the Palazzo: the Medici emblem of three feathers in a diamond ring is set in stone beneath the vase of lilies.

36. ABOVE *Synagoga, c.* 1230
Stone (Strasburg Munster)

One of the finest figures in German Gothic sculpture, Synagoga stands in the south transept of Strasburg Munster and, together with an accompanying statue of Ecclesia, it shows magnificently the elegant S shape and the heavy, folded drapery of High Gothic art. Synagoga personified the Old Testament, Ecclesia the New, and Synagoga's blindfold is a symbol of her ignorance of the New.

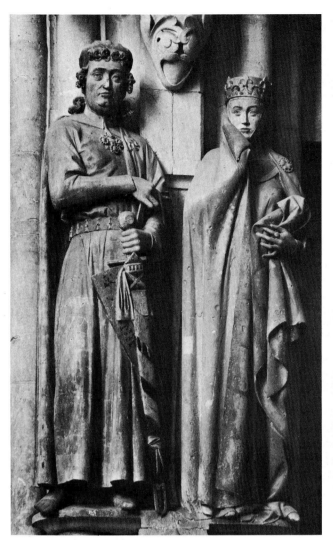 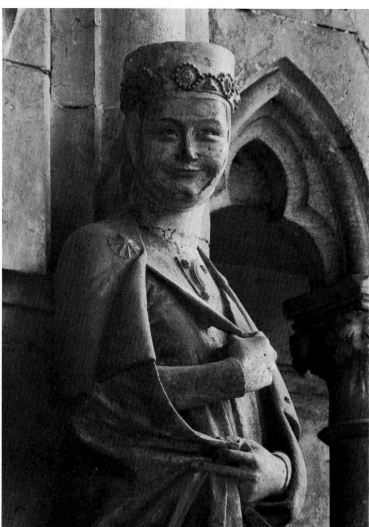

37. ABOVE LEFT *Woman with a Cloak, c.* 1250–60
Stone (Naumburg Cathedral)

This startlingly life-like portrait at Naumburg in Saxony is of Uta, the wife of Ekkhard, one of the
founders of the thirteenth-century Cathedral. It is one of several portraits of noblemen
and women responsible for founding the Cathedral, which are arrayed along the responds
inside the choir. They were sculpted long after their deaths, but the artist has given each one an
individual personality.

38. ABOVE RIGHT *Smiling Woman, c.* 1250–60
Stone (Naumburg Cathedral)

Sculpted by the same hand as the *Woman with a Cloak*, the same unusual treatment can be seen in
the face of this comely, smiling woman. Little is known about the sculptor, but his artistic
development can be traced through France and Germany, culminating in his work at Naumburg in
the 1250s and 60s. It was here that he introduced new elements into his figures, a dramatic
expression and a solidity of structure that sets them apart from the mainstream of Gothic sculpture.

39. OPPOSITE Dieric Bouts, *Virgin and Child*
Oil on panel (Bargello, Florence)

The most beautiful of all Bouts' pictures of the Virgin and Child. The figures are presented as if
they were sculpture, and it is possible that Bouts had seen the works of Donatello when he was
in Italy.

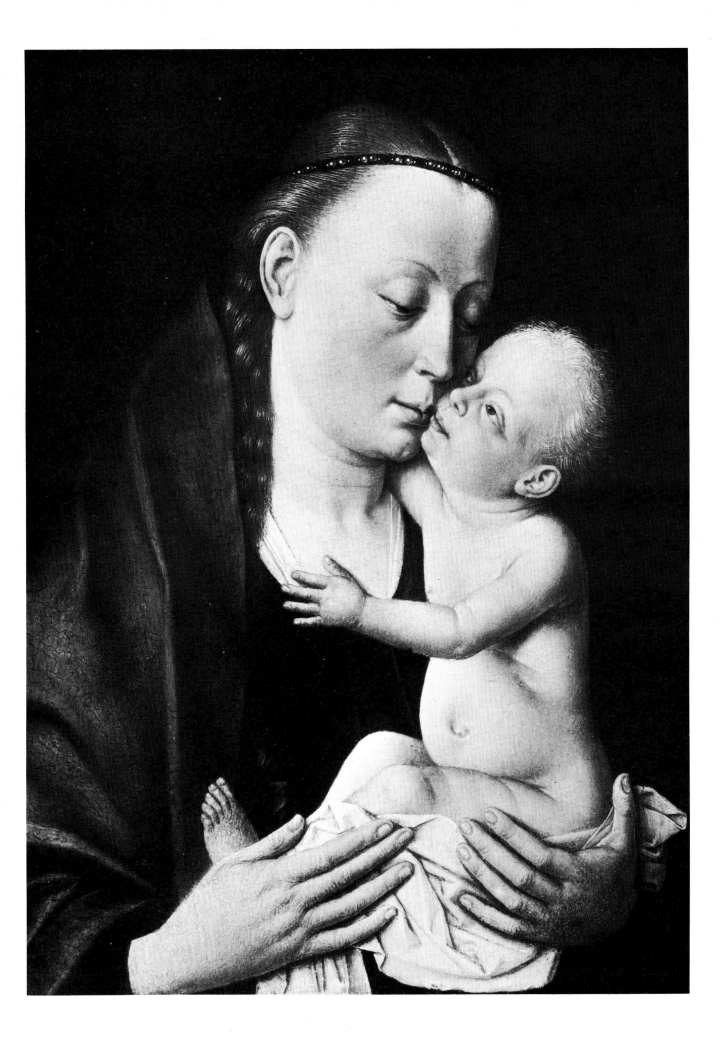

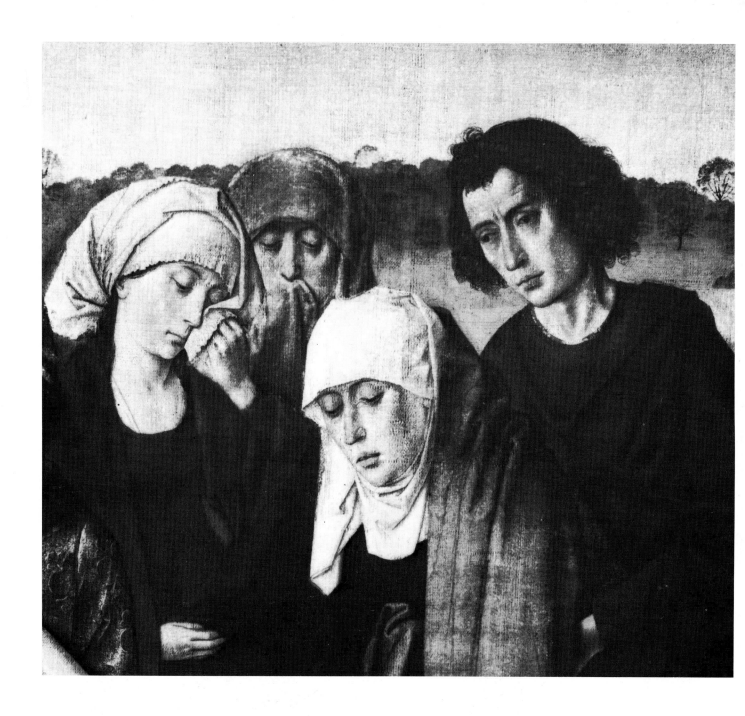

40. ABOVE Dieric Bouts, *Entombment* (detail)
Tempera on flax (National Gallery, London)

These intense, pale faces seem suspended in time and space, their expressions of grief frozen for ever. Bouts, like many northern painters, took a miniaturist's care in the modelling of his figures, which, as in this case, gives his pictures intimacy and naturalism.

41. OPPOSITE Lucas Cranach the Elder, *Cupid Complaining to Venus*, after 1552
Wood (National Gallery, London)

As Court Painter to the Electors of Saxony at Wittenburg, Cranach painted many nudes in response to the demands of the sophisticated court. His females are contemporary women, often, as in this case, bedecked with fantastic props such as large, plumed hats and enormous necklaces, which accentuate their nakedness and their slender, elegant eroticism.

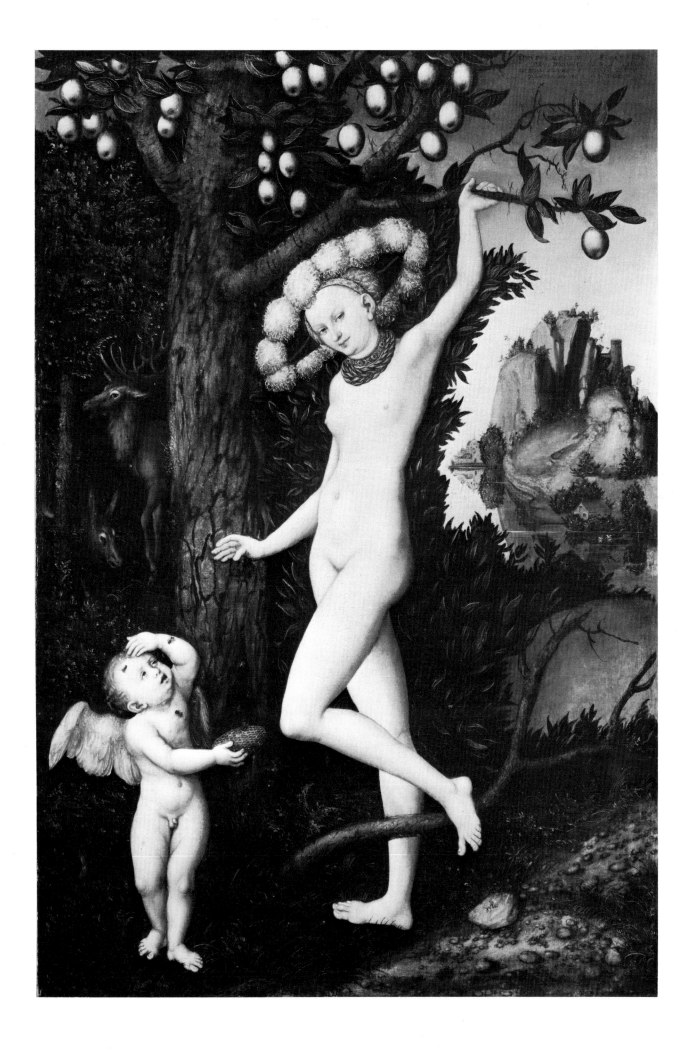

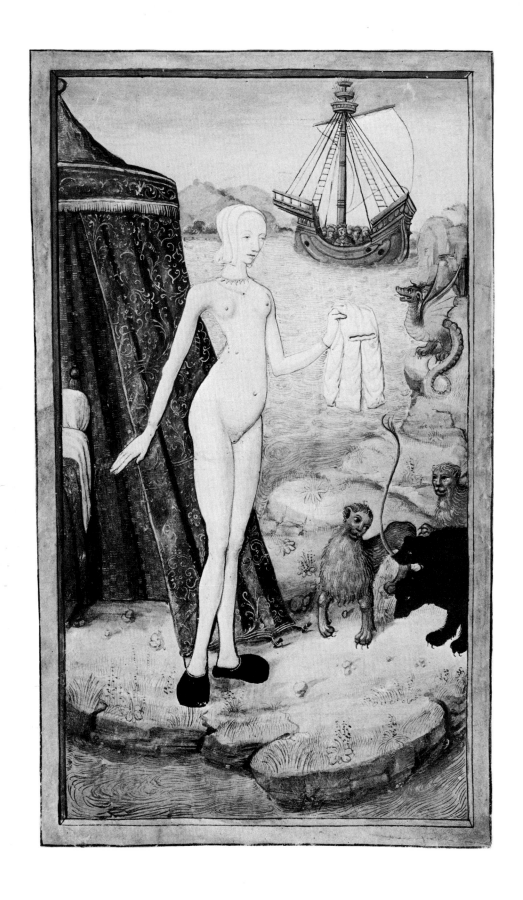

42. *Ariadne on Naxos*, Illustration for Ovid's Heriodes
Vellum (Bibliothèque Nationale, Paris)

An anonymous French painter's illustration of Ariadne deserted by Theseus on the island of Naxos,
a place populated by monsters. She is naked except for her hat, jewels and rather surprising
bathing clogs.

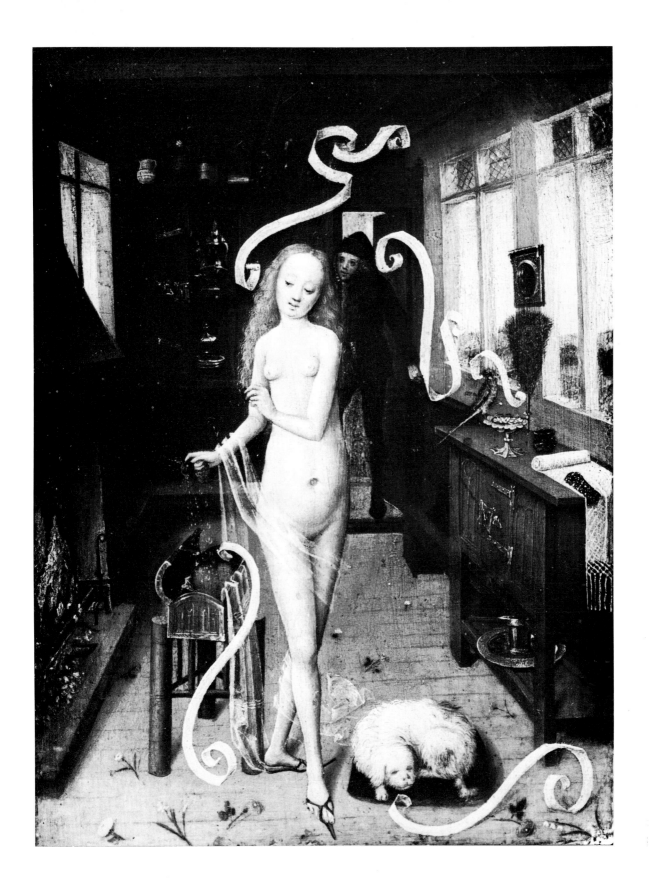

43. The Master of Niederrheim, *The Charm of Love*
Oil on canvas (Leipzig Museum)

Unlike *Ariadne on Naxos*, this example of northern fantasy has all the attributes of allure that Lucas
Cranach was later to perfect. The scene is set in a comfortable interior, with a blazing fire reflecting
on objects in the room, and catching the light of the jewels in the sorceress's hand. She seems to be
well aware of her beauty, and confident in her spells.

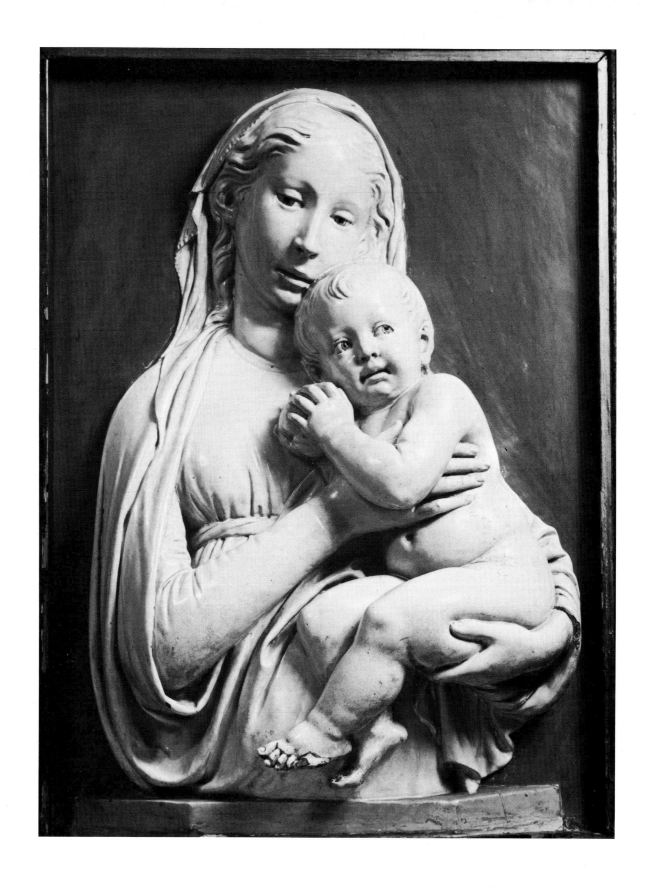

44. Luca della Robbia, *Madonna della Mela*, c. 1450
Glazed terracotta (Bargello, Florence)

The medium of glazed terracotta perfectly conveys the sweetness of this Madonna's face. Luca della
Robbia used his discovery in a large number of architectural and decorative reliefs, often
contrasting the milky whiteness of his figures with a dramatic blue background or coloured
garlands of vegetation, producing a cameo-like effect.

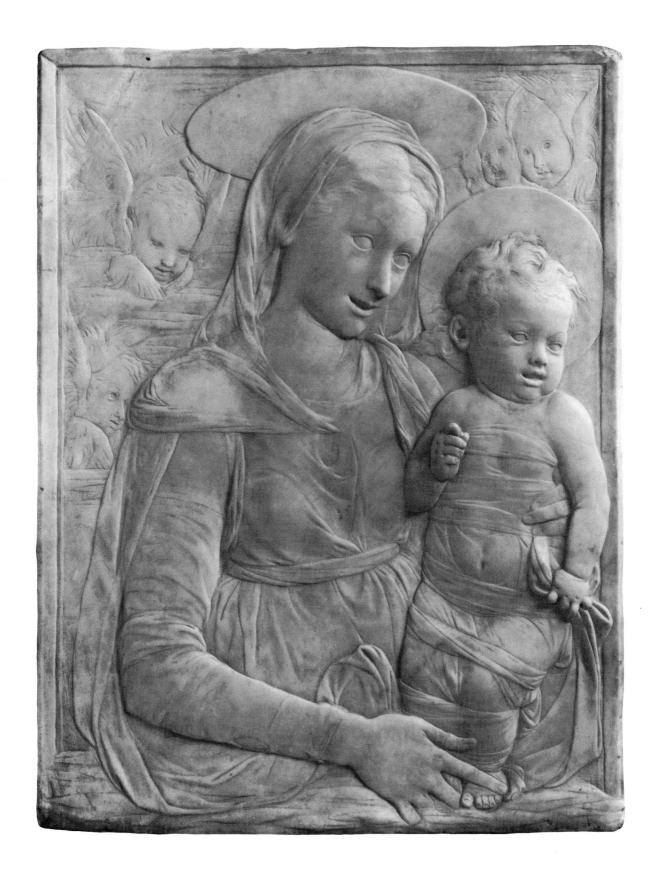

45. Desiderio da Settignano, *Virgin and Child*, *c.* 1460
Marble (Philadelphia Museum of Art: The W. P. Wilstach Collection)

Desiderio da Settignano is well known for this type of relief, depicting the Virgin as a smiling young mother playing with her child. Within the depth of less than one inch, he has managed to convey several levels of perspective, and has achieved a quite remarkable variation of texture. The relief is believed to have been housed in a small chapel attached to the Hospitale di Santa Maria Nuova in Florence.

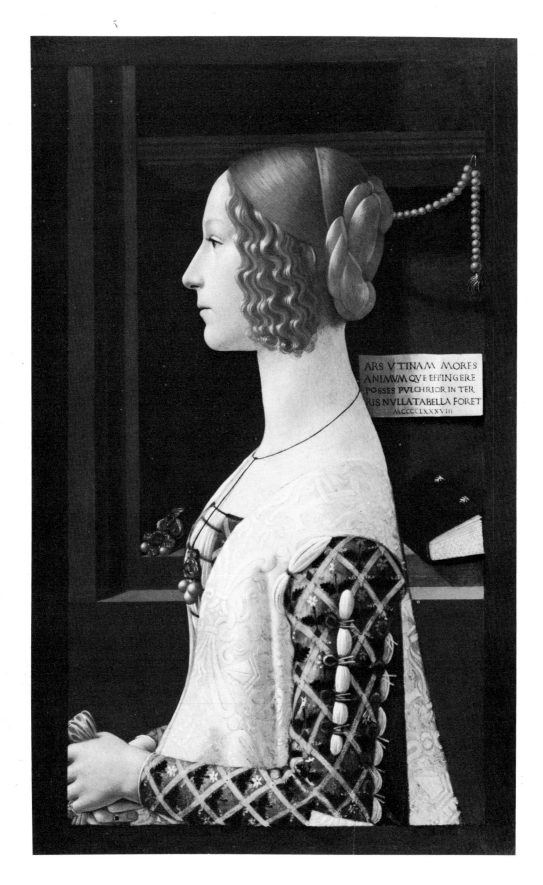

46. Domenico Ghirlandaio, *Giovanna Tornabuoni*, after 1488
Panel (Thyssen Collection, Lugano)

Profile portraits were extremely popular in fifteenth-century Italy. This young girl was painted posthumously on the instructions of her father-in-law, and the composition was copied from family frescos that Ghirlandaio had completed a few years before. The artst is well known for his precise attention to detail, which is admirably shown in this formal portrait.

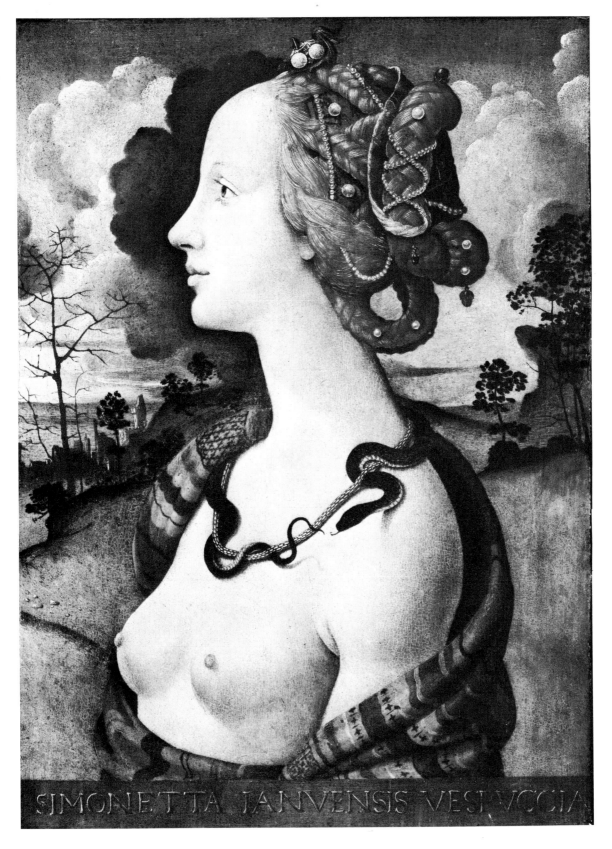

SIMONETTA IANVENSIS VESPVCCIA

47. Piero di Cosimo, *Simonetta Vespucci*
Panel (Musée Condé, Chantilly)

The poet Poliziano spoke of Simonetta's 'winding ringlets of golden hair', and in this portrait Piero di Cosimo had made decorative use of her elaborate plaits interwoven with pearls. Simonetta was a famous beauty in Florence at the time of Lorenzo the Magnificent, and attracted the amorous attentions of his brother, Giuliano. Her beauty was short lived: she died of consumption at only twenty-three.

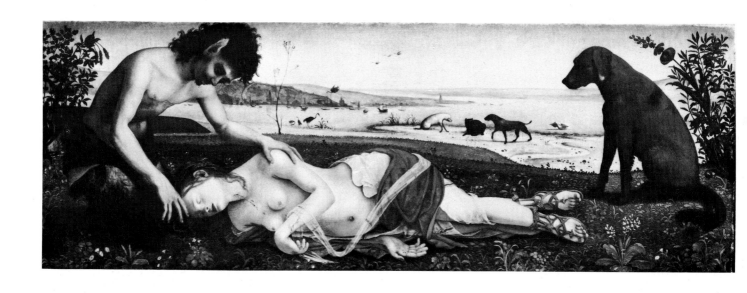

48. ABOVE Piero di Cosimo, *A Mythological Subject*
Wood (National Gallery, London)

The subject matter of this painting remains unsolved, although it probably illustrates a classical myth or Renaissance poem. Vasari writes that Piero di Cosimo's observations of nature sometimes 'drove him quite out of his mind with delight', and his pleasure is evident here in the painting of plants and flowers and in the attitude of the grieving dog. The same powers of acute observation are apparent in his delicate rendering of the dying nymph.

49. OPPOSITE Leonardo da Vinci, *Portrait of a Lady with an Ermine (Cecilia Gallerani)*, 1485–90
Oil on panel (Czartoryski Museum, Cracow)

Cecilia Gallerani was born about 1465, the daughter of a Milanese nobleman who was Ambassador to Florence. Later, as mistress of Ludovico Sforza, she reigned over the Milanese court, and it was there that Leonardo painted her. The ermine she holds in her arms not only mirrors her intense alertness but is also a subtle pun on her name: the Greek word for ermine plays on Gallerani. The picture found its way into the collection of Prince Adam Czartoryski at the end of the eighteenth century.

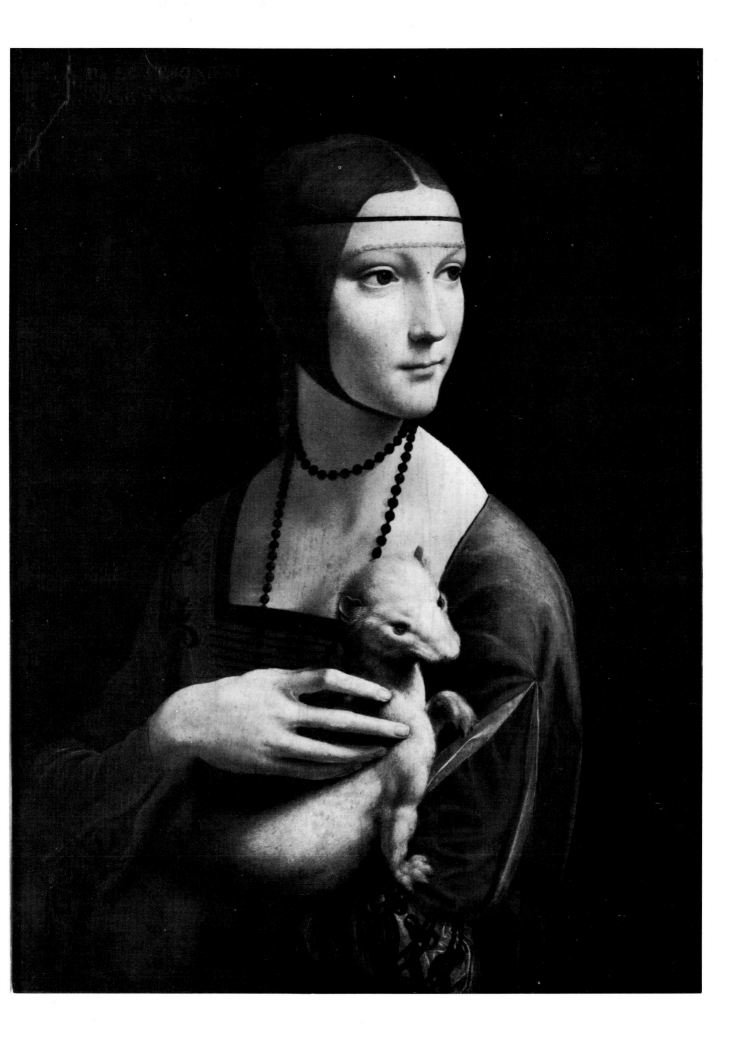

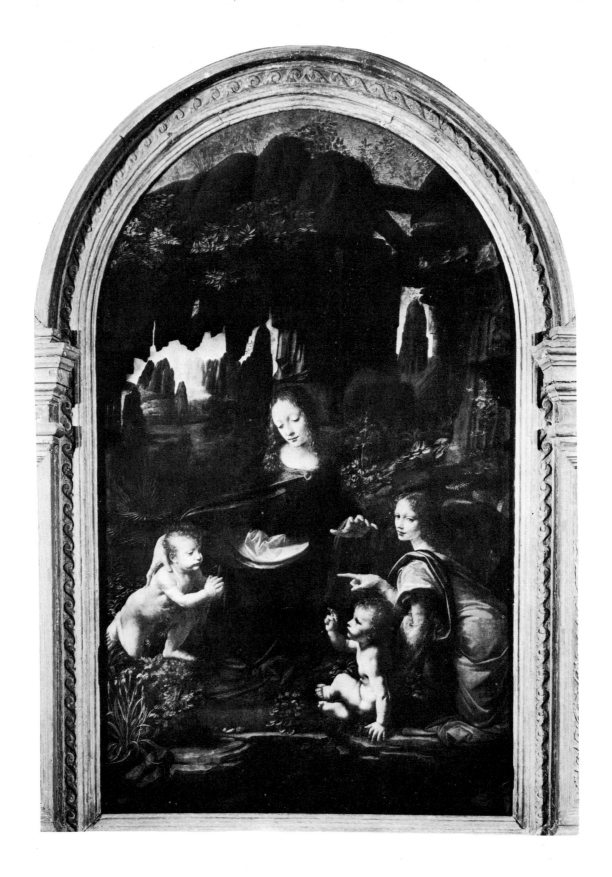

50. Leonardo da Vinci, *Virgin of the Rocks*, 1483–6
Oil on canvas (Louvre, Paris)

This is almost certainly the picture recorded in Leonardo's inventory as 'unfinished' when he took it from Florence to Milan in 1483. It was subsequently worked on and may have become part of an altarpiece in Milan. It was sold to the King of France, and taken to Fontainebleau, where it is mentioned in an inventory of 1623. At some point a replica, in which Leonardo painted some details, was made in his studio, and is now in the National Gallery, London.

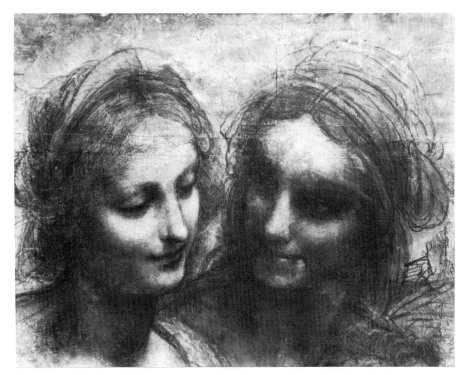

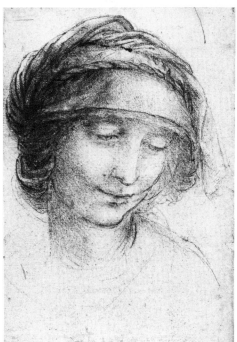

51. TOP Leonardo da Vinci, *The Virgin and Child with St Anne and St John the Baptist* (detail), *c.* 1498
Black chalk heightened with white (National Gallery, London)

The enigmatic expression of St Anne contrasts with the maternal tenderness and simplicity of the face of the Virgin. They are both imbued with such grace and loveliness that they must surely rank as Leonardo's most haunting creations.

52. ABOVE Leonardo da Vinci, *Head of St Anne*
Charcoal (By Gracious Permission of H.M. the Queen, Windsor Castle Library)

The same beautiful expression belongs to the St Anne drawing at Windsor Castle.

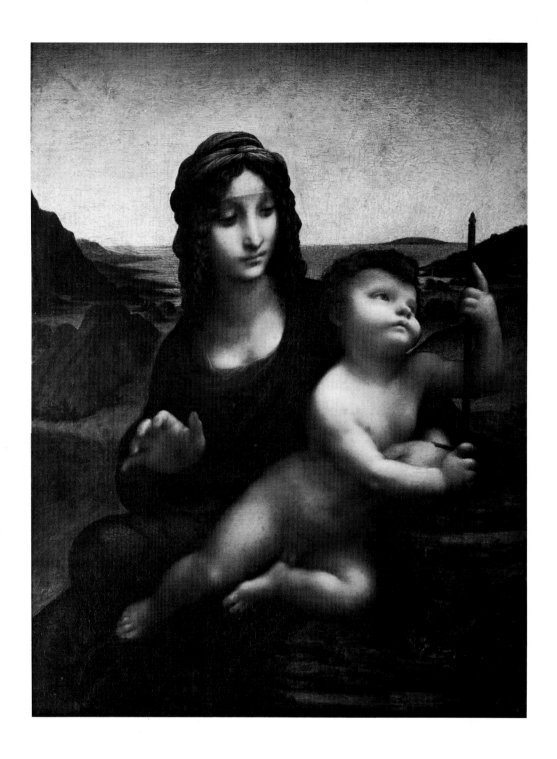

53. ABOVE Leonardo da Vinci, *Madonna with the Yard Winder, c.* 1500–10
Oil on canvas (Duke of Buccleuch and Queensberry Collection, Boughton)

Painted for Florimond Robertet, the Secretary of State for Louis XII, this picture symbolizes the Passion of Christ. The Christ Child gazes at the cross-shaped yarn winder and holds it tightly, while the Madonna anxiously tries to take it from him. Leonardo's gentle, melancholy women were to be copied time and again by lesser artists in an attempt to recreate their particular beauty.

54. OPPOSITE Piero del Pollaiuolo, *Portrait of a Young Woman, c.* 1475
Tempera on wood (Poldi Pezzoli, Milan)

As interest in classical art grew, artists emulated the profile portraits of Greeks and Romans on coins and medals. This charming, fresh-faced sitter has a remarkably modern appearance, despite her plucked hairline and bejewelled hair, and her picture can be numbered among the first society portraits.

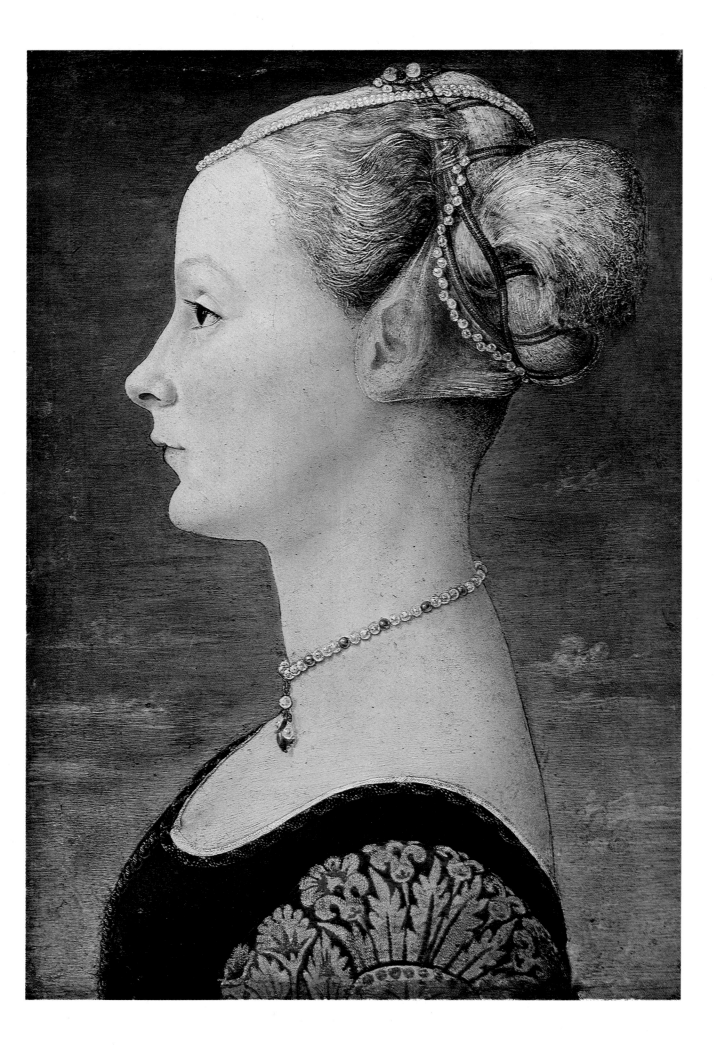

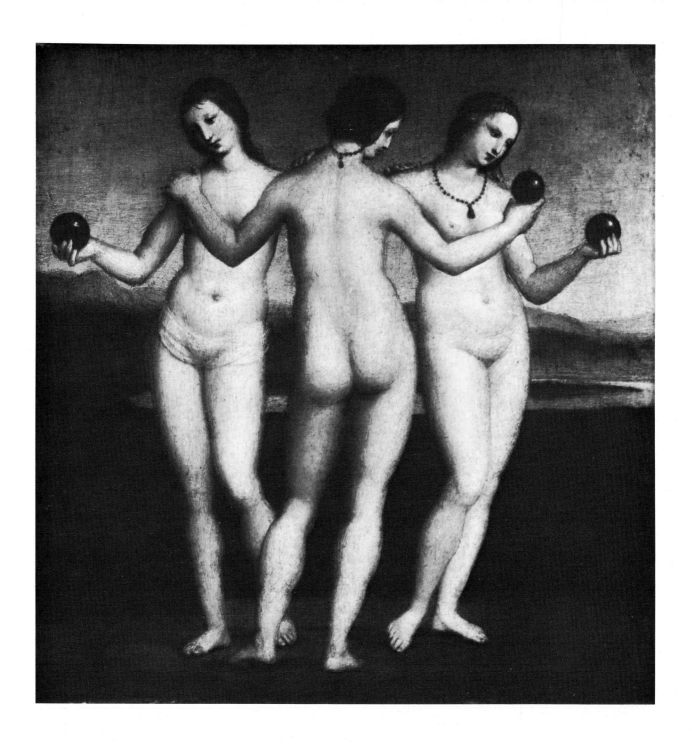

55. ABOVE Raffaello Sanzio (Raphael), *The Three Graces*, 1504–5
Oil on panel (Musée Condé, Chantilly)

Raphael was brought up in the harmonious and cultured court of Federigo Montefeltro, Duke of
Urbino, where his father was Court Painter. His intrinsic sense of proportion and form owe their
beginnings to that magnificent palace. The small frieze-like group at Chantilly is probably taken
from a classical model which has now disappeared. The motif was rare in classical times, and the
few surviving examples lack the fullness of form of Raphael's painting.

56. OPPOSITE Raffaello Sanzio (Raphael), *La Donna Velata*, 1516
Oil on canvas (Pitti Palace, Florence)

This late portrait is probably that of Raphael's mistress, known to us as La Fornarina. He painted
her many times, and often insisted that she be near him while he worked. Vasari relates that 'he was
indeed a very amorous man with a great fondness for women'.

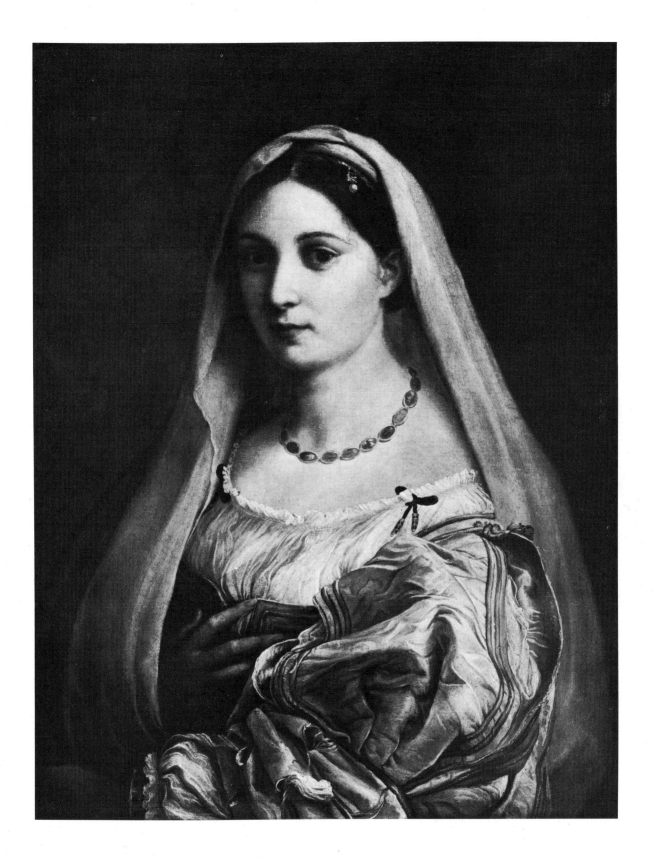

57. OVERLEAF Sandro Botticelli, *Primavera*, *c.* 1477–8
Tempera on wood (Uffizi, Florence)

The *Primavera* was painted as part of a commission for Lorenzo di Pierfrancesco de Medici, a second cousin of the great Lorenzo, and was housed in his villa at Castello. The meaning of the allegory is arguable, but what is certain is its relation to Neo-Platonic thought, popular in Florence at the time and preached by Marsilio Ficino and the poet Poliziano. Botticelli's concept of beauty was much admired by his contempories and enjoyed a renewed popularity under the Pre-Raphaelites in nineteenth-century England.

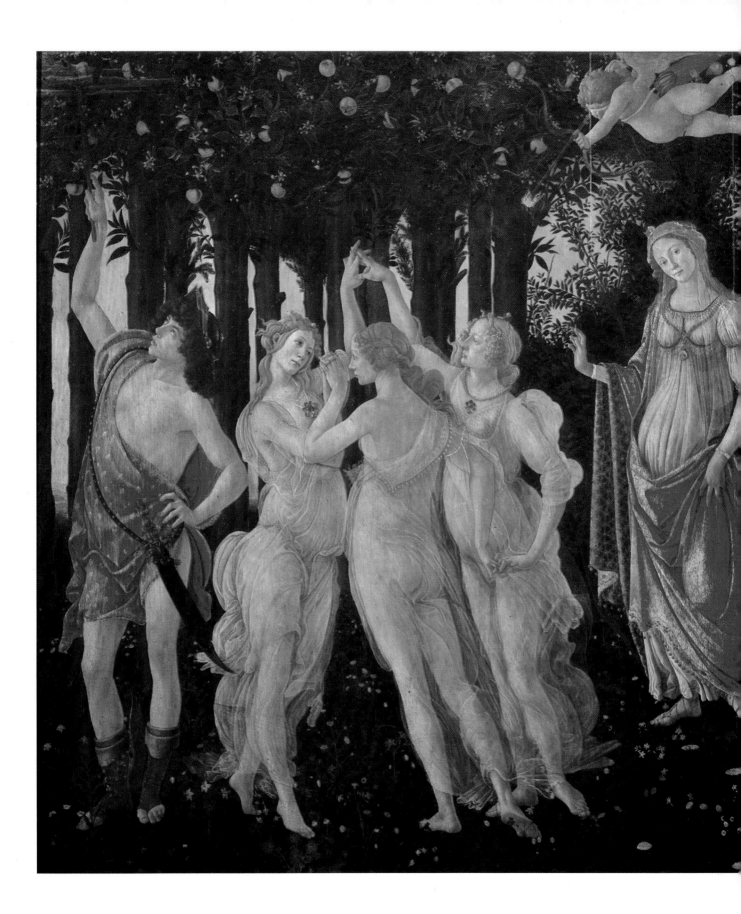

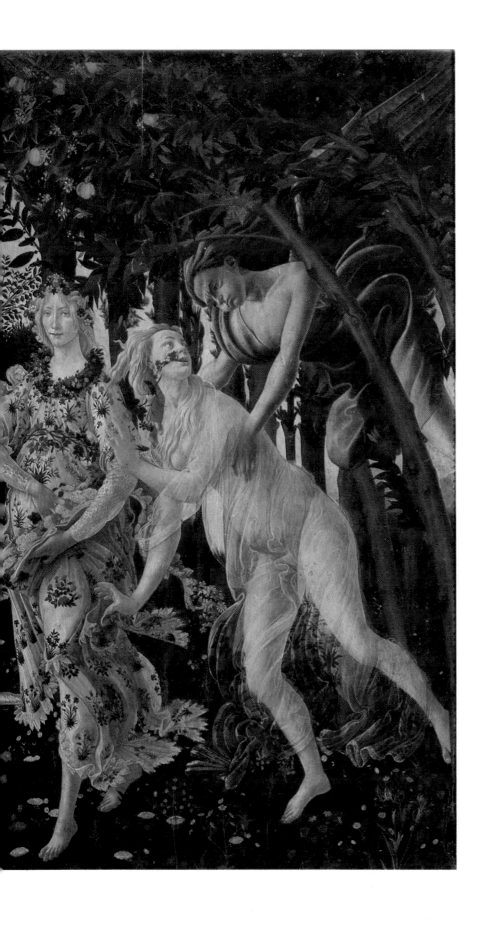

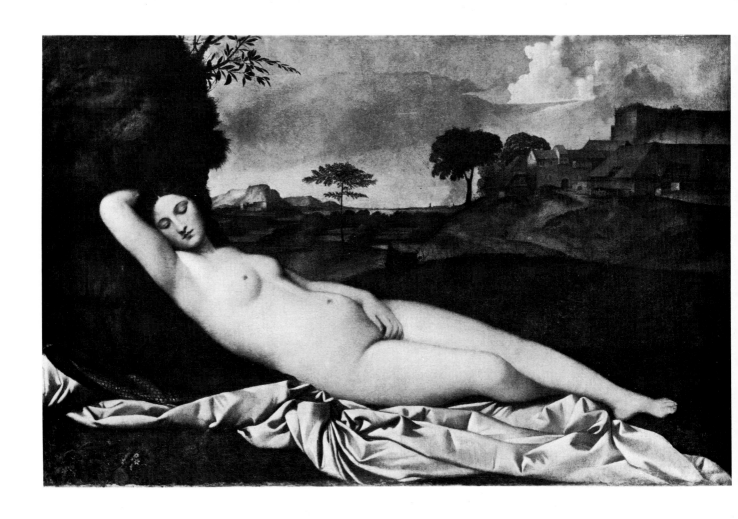

58. ABOVE Giorgione, *Sleeping Venus (The Dresden Venus)*
Oil on canvas (Gemaldegalerie, Dresden)

The reclining nude seems to have no precedent in classical art, and with the *Sleeping Venus*
Giorgione initiated a genre that was to become immensely popular. There is an element of the
Gothic style in the attenuated pose and rounded stomach of this elegant Venus, whose expression is
one of pure innocence without a trace of immodesty.

59. OPPOSITE ABOVE Tiziano Vecelli (Titian), *Venus of Urbino*, 1538
Oil on canvas (Uffizi, Florence)

Clearly the *Venus of Urbino* owes her origins to Giorgione's *Sleeping Venus*. But this reclining nude
is totally different in feeling. Titian has placed her not in a landscape but in a domestic interior
surrounded by creature comforts, and her gaze is sensual and inviting.

60. OPPOSITE BELOW Tiziano Vecelli (Titian), *Venus with the Organist*, c. 1550
Oil on canvas (Prado, Madrid)

This is one of a series of paintings Titian executed on the theme of music and art: perhaps a
reference to the Neo-Platonic argument as to whether beauty is better appreciated through the eye
or the ear. But the beauty displayed here has an almost over-blown quality, and its full frontal
attack on the senses lacks some of the charm of his earlier beauties.

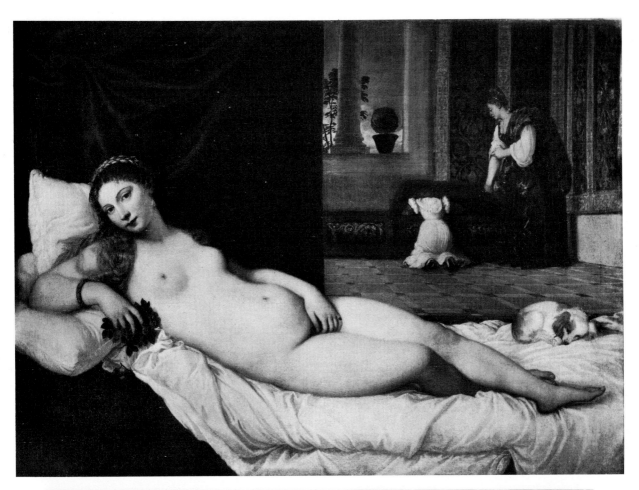

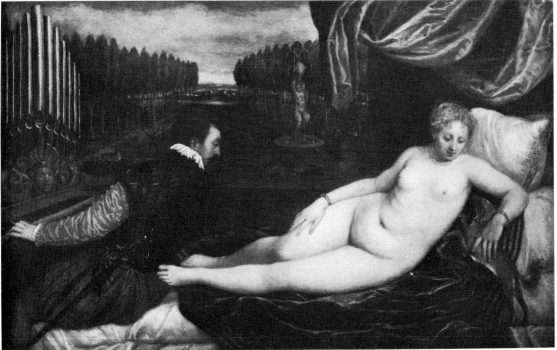

61. OVERLEAF Sandro Botticelli, *Birth of Venus* (detail), *c.* 1478
Tempera on wood (Uffizi, Florence)

The *Birth of Venus* and the *Primavera* were part of the same commission for Lorenzo di
Pierfrancesco de Medici. An intricate blend of pagan philosophies and Christianity inspired
this figure (modelled by Simonetta Vespucci), which combines a nude Venus with the ideal of the
Virgin Mary as the source of 'divine love'.

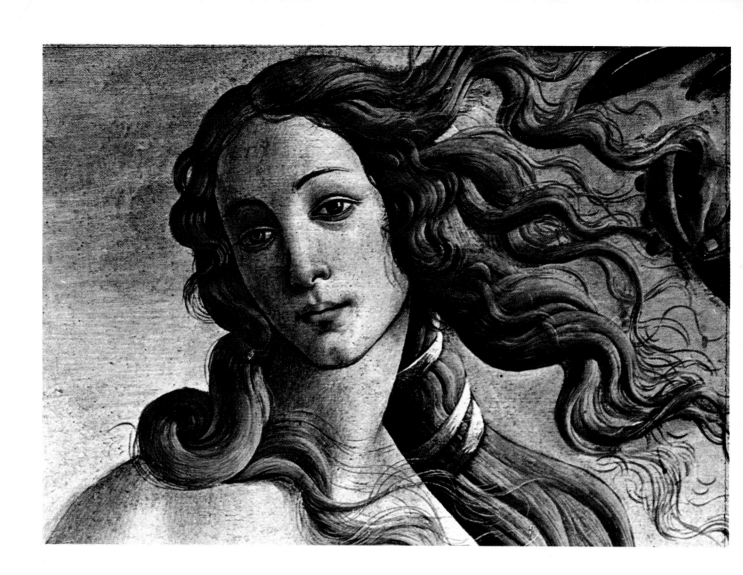

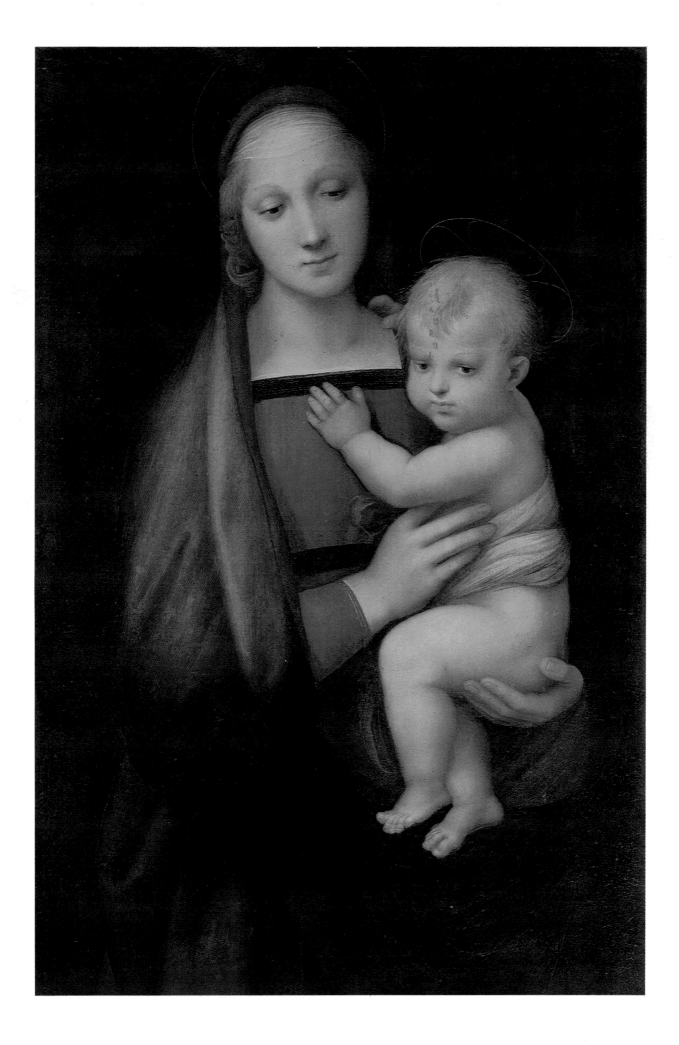

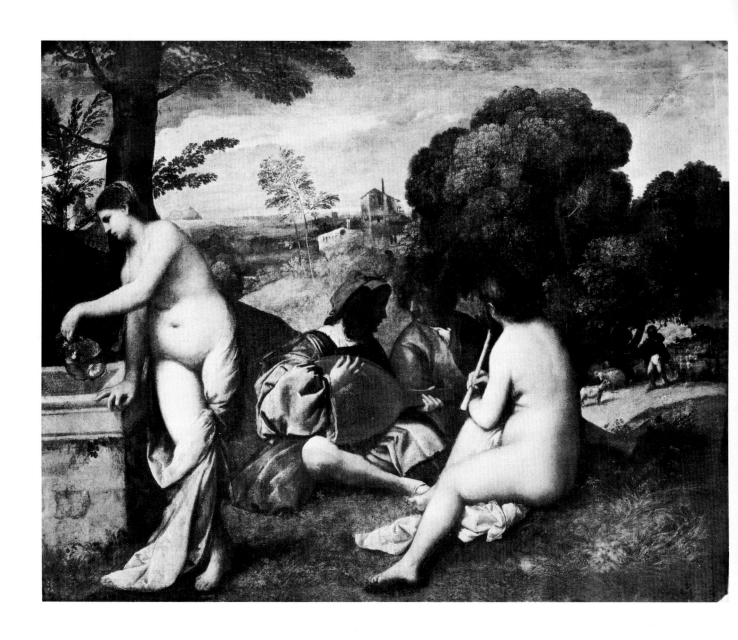

62. PRECEDING PAGE Raffaello Sanzio (Raphael), *Granduca Madonna*, 1504
Oil on panel (Pitti Palace, Florence)

It is perhaps in this painting of the Madonna and Child that Raphael achieves his ultimate
expression of beauty. The Madonna's calm, harmonious face has become the traditional model
for the perfect image of the Virgin. Raphael said of his work that he followed '*una certa idea*'
and not an earthly inspiration.

63. ABOVE Giorgione, *Concert Châmpetre*
Oil on canvas (Louvre, Paris)

The theme of the nude in a landscape recurs in this unusual concert scene, which could be
interpreted as an allegory of the senses, and was to be echoed three hundred years later by Manet.
Unlike Manet, Giorgione has painted his figures as an integral part of the Arcadian landscape,
unselfconscious and apparently unaware that they are being observed.

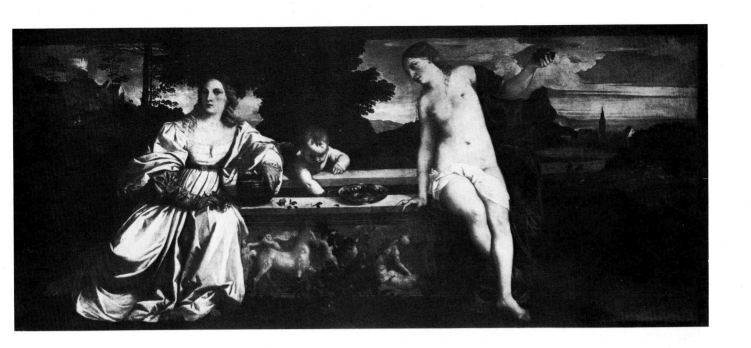

64. ABOVE Tiziano Vecelli (Titian), *Sacred and Profane Love, c.* 1515
Oil on canvas (Borghese Gallery, Rome)

The title and meaning of this painting are uncertain, but it is thought that the two women, naked and clothed, represent the different aspects of love. Titian, during his long life, was to be wooed by kings and princes, and fêted by every court in Europe, but his inspirations for beauty remained the golden-haired women of Veneto.

65. OVERLEAF LEFT Tiziano Vecelli (Titian), *Venus Anadyomene, c.* 1520
Oil on canvas (National Gallery of Scotland, Edinburgh)

The subject of the isolated nude, bereft of a mythological or Neo-Platonic setting, is very rare indeed before the nineteenth century. This Venus, however, is one of the most complete expressions of the nude for nude's sake outside antique art. Why Titian should have broken away from tradition in this way is unclear. One hypothesis is that, in order to preserve it, he was asked to copy one of the figures that he and Giorgione had frescoed in the Fondaco de Tedeschi in Venice.

66. OVERLEAF RIGHT Lorenzo Lotto, *Triumph of Chastity, c.* 1530
Oil on canvas (Pallavicini Collection, Rome)

The clear colours and cold skin tones in this work portray a purely intellectual sensuality, but at the same time, the fine modelling of the face and body of Venus is in the Venetian tradition of Titian and Giorgione. It is interesting to note the objects that Lotto has included in this allegory – the ermine, dove and shells – as symbols of Chastity and Venus. The painting was acquired by the Pallavicini family in the late eighteenth-century.

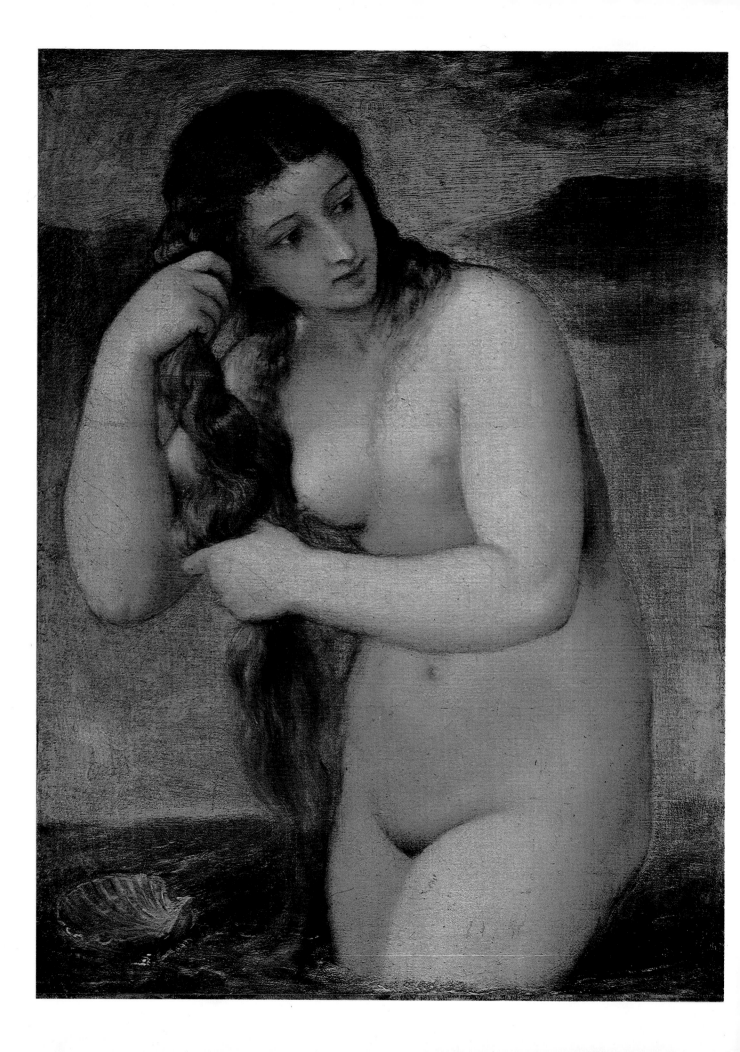

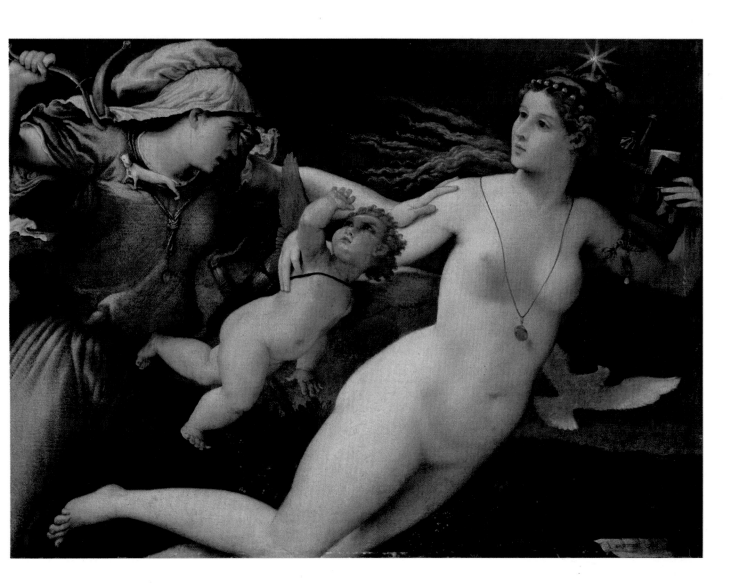

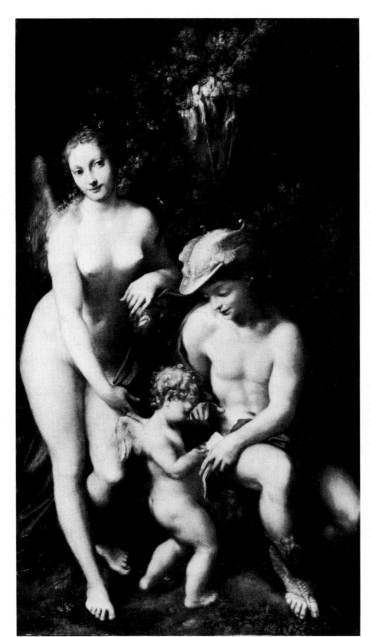 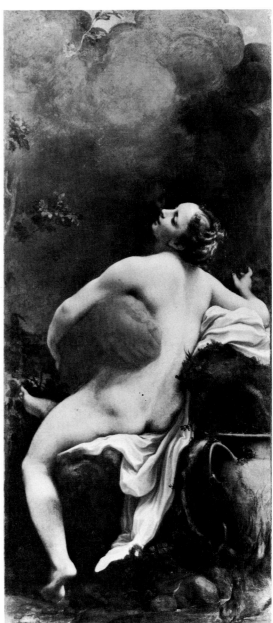

67. ABOVE LEFT Antonio Correggio, *The School of Love (Mercury instructing Cupid before Venus)*, *c.* 1628
Oil on canvas (National Gallery, London)

The mythological subject of Cupid, so often the teacher of love, brought by Venus, his mother, to Mercury for a reading lesson allows Correggio to be overt in his expression of sensuality. He achieves this by giving a rounded fullness to the *sfumato* figures. X-ray photographs have shown that the faces of Venus and Mercury were first painted in different positions.

68. ABOVE RIGHT Antonio Correggio, *Io*, *c.* 1531
Oil on canvas (Kunsthistorisches Museum, Vienna)

Io is from a series of pictures depicting the Loves of Jove, commissioned by Federigo II Gonzaga for the coronation of Charles V at Bologna in 1530. A voluptuous nymph, seen here in the arms of Jove, who is surrounded by mist, tilts her head upwards and back to receive the god's embraces. The influence of the antique is evident not only in the choice of subject matter but also in the large urn in the foreground. The picture's characteristic lightness and grace, together with its sense of mystery, are the factors which have labelled Correggio proto-Baroque.

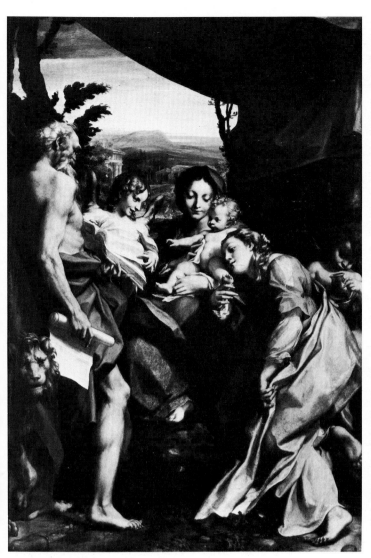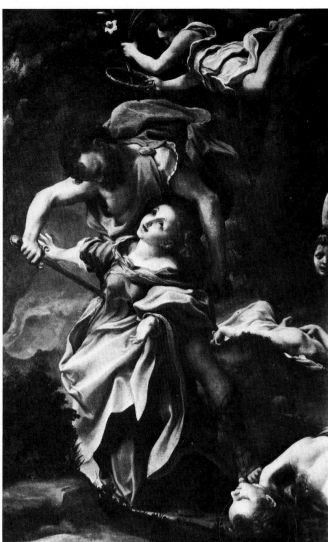

69. ABOVE LEFT Antonio Correggio, *Madonna of St Jerome*, 1527–8
Oil on wood (Pinacoteca, Parma)

The concave grouping and strong diagonal movement of this large painting give a sense of energy
to an otherwise peaceful scene, and the tender concern of the faces creates a unity of mood. This
painting, which is also known as *Il Giorno*, was closely followed by a complementary *Adoration of
the Shepherds*, known as *Il Notte*.

70. ABOVE RIGHT Antonio Correggio, *Martyrdom of St Placido and St Flavia* (detail), *c.* 1524–36
Oil on canvas (Pinacoteca, Parma)

The figures in Correggio's *Martyrdom* have sensuous, rhythmic artificiality, and, despite the pain
that is being inflicted on them, expressions of pure ecstasy. The violence is complemented by the
mannered poses of the saints, and the whole design manipulated into ornament as elaborate as any
in Maniera.

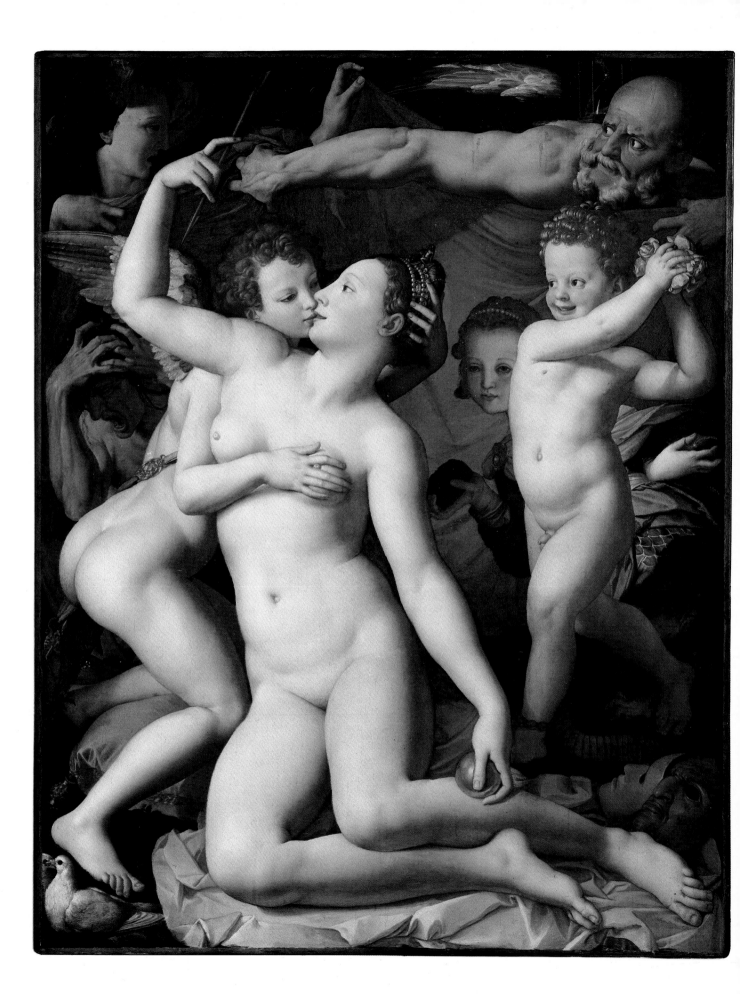

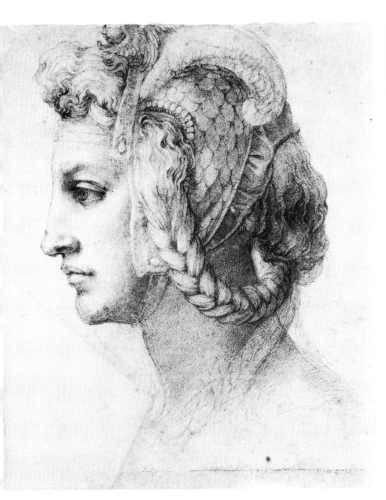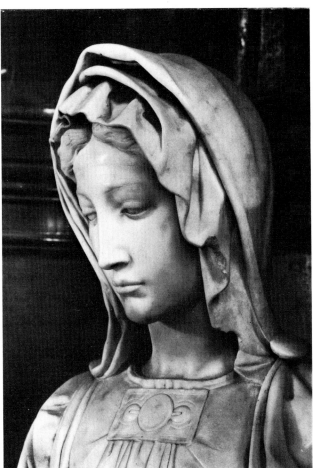

71. OPPOSITE Agnolo Bronzino. *Venus, Cupid, Time and Folly, c.* 1540–60
Oil on wood (National Gallery, London)

This exotic allegory, based on a complex verbal allegory of the Passions of Love, was painted for Cosimo I de Medici, who later presented it to François I of France. The figures have been turned into a sculptured relief, but they are nonetheless intensely erotic. Bronzino was a pupil of Pontormo and a great admirer of Michelangelo, yet his art has its own peculiar intensity and feeling of cold abstraction. He took Mannerism to a realm of polished decadence previously unknown.

72. ABOVE LEFT Michelangelo Buonarroti, *Testa Divina, c.* 1520
Drawing (British Museum, London)

The young Michelangelo was allowed to study in the gardens of the Palazzo Medici, and there he made careful studies of antique sculptures, a classical influence which appears in the group of drawings known as *Teste Divine*: the earliest was executed *c.* 1520. He achieved a contemporary ideal in the woman's classical features, but the most striking element of the work is her ornate and fantastic head-dress. The drawing is a compact demonstration of refinement and imagination.

73. ABOVE RIGHT Michelangelo Buonarroti, *Bruges Madonna* (detail), 1501
Marble (Bruges Cathedral)

This Madonna was carved by Michelangelo while he was still a young man, but, although the subject is a familiar one, he gives it new and deeper meaning. Instead of her usual smile, she has an expression of contemplative melancholy, as if she foresees her son's fate.

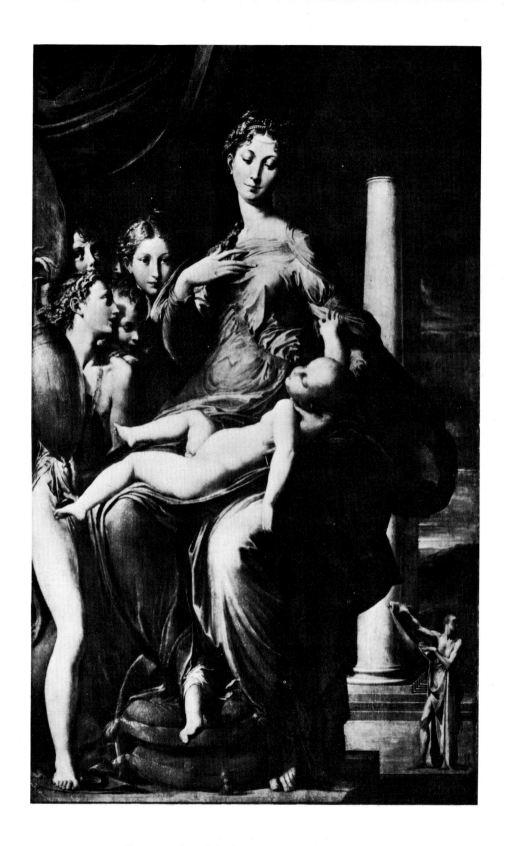

74. Francesco Parmigianino, *Madonna del Col Lungo*, 1535
Oil on canvas (Uffizi, Florence)

Parmigianino was a pupil of Correggio, and his painting has a refined, intellectual elegance in its composition, brilliance of colour and affectation of gesture. *The Madonna del Col Lungo*, begun in 1534 but never finished, portrays a tall, slender Madonna of porcelain delicacy, whose attitude would be more suitable to a pagan goddess than to the Mother of Christ. No other sixteenth-century painting goes so far in its transformation of the human form into an image of artificial grace. Despite the fact that the figures are elongated to the point of absurdity, there is a reference to the calm classicism of the High Renaissance in the column in the background.

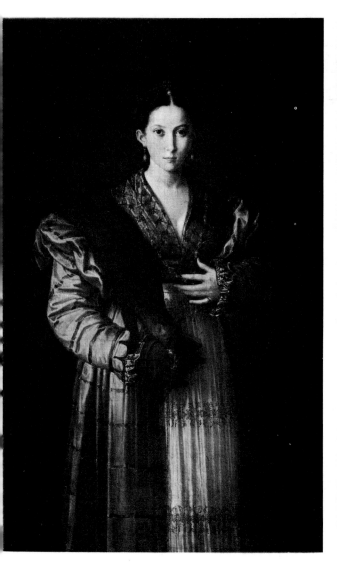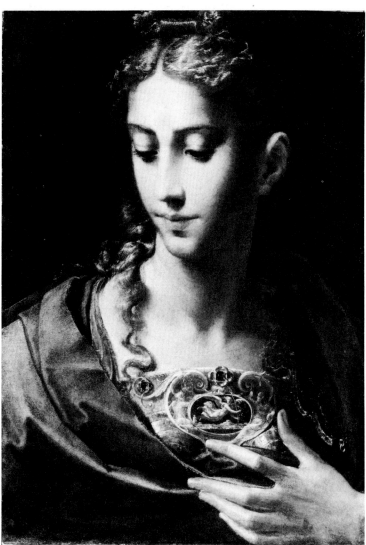

75. ABOVE LEFT Francesco Parmigianino, *Antea*
Oil on canvas (Museo Nazionale, Naples)

Nothing is known of the beautiful sitter except her name. She was evidently a lady of high fashion, and is represented, as usual in such portraits, in her finest dress.

76. ABOVE RIGHT Francesco Parmigianino, *Minerva*, c. 1528
Oil on canvas (By Gracious Permission of H.M. the Queen)

Fancy 'portraits' of this kind were in fashion in Italian art in the early sixteenth-century, and did not represent any particular goddess. I can see no reason why this was identified with Minerva, none of whose attributes are apparent. But the title has become accepted.

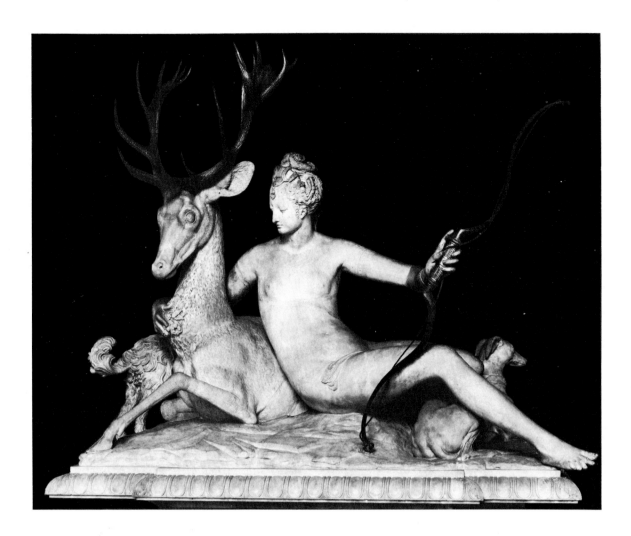

77. ABOVE School of Fontainebleau, *Diane d'Anet*, after 1555
Marble (Louvre, Paris)

Called the *Diane d'Anet* because it stood in a courtyard at Diane de Poitier's chateau at Anet, this
Diana has the elegance and decorativeness that only the French seem to have captured: a blend of
the northern and the Mediterranean spirit. It was once believed that this Diana was the likeness of
Diane de Poitiers, but the theory has now been rejected on the grounds that the face is too stylized
and too dissimilar from portraits known to be hers.

78. OPPOSITE ABOVE School of Fontainebleau, *Diane de Poitiers*, c. 1550
Oil on canvas (Kunstmuseum, Basle)

The famous mistress of Henri II of France is seen here at her toilette, a thin gauze veil covering her
shoulders. There is an overt sensuality in the hand touching her breast and in the coupled figures
beneath her image in the mirror. This stylishness is typical of the Mannerist School of
Fontainebleau, which became the main centre of Italian Renaissance ideas in northern Europe.

79. OPPOSITE BELOW Pellegrino Tibaldi, *Ulysses Shipwrecked* (ceiling decoration), begun 1533
Fresco (Palazzo Poggi, Bologna)

In the vigorous style and alarming perspective of Tibaldi's work, Mannerism is taken to its farthest
extreme. He based his studies on Michelangelo, and blended them with the elegance of
Parmigianino and Nicolo dell'Abbate, who disseminated the Mannerist ideas in France by working
at Fontainebleau. The tortuous and extravagant postures are certainly very daring, but they
sounded the funeral march for Mannerism.

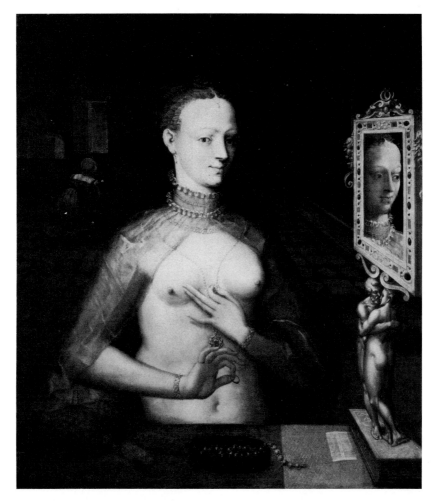

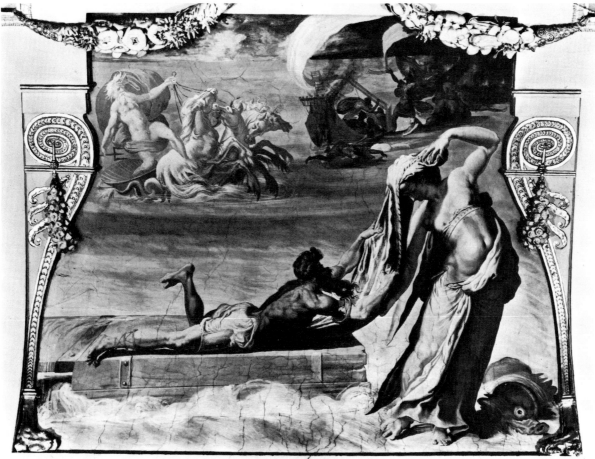

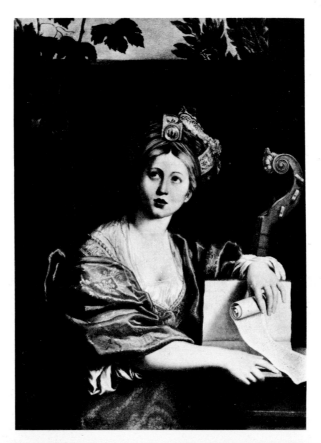

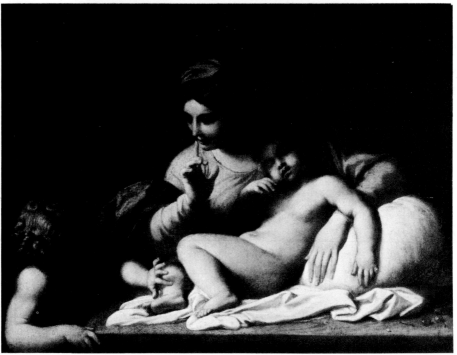

80. TOP Domenichino, *Sibyl*, *c.* 1617
Oil on canvas (Borghese Gallery, Rome)

Domenichino was one of the foremost pupils of the Carracci brothers. He helped Annibale with the
decorations in the Farnese Palace, and worked in both Rome and Naples. But as the years passed,
his High Renaissance style, learned from the Carracci, went out of fashion, and the more exuberant
Baroque of Lanfranco and Pietro da Cortona took over as the popular style. However, his series of
paintings of sibyls and prophetesses, of which this is one, seemed never to lose their appeal.

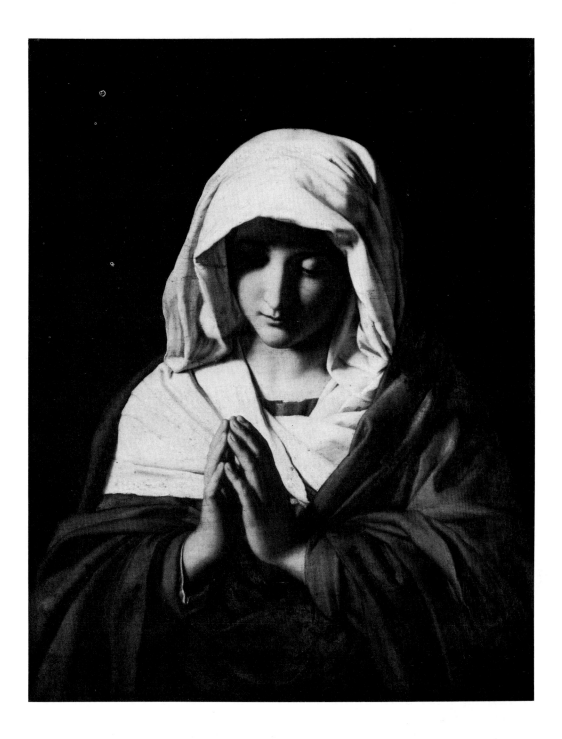

81. OPPOSITE BELOW Annibale Carracci, *Madonna and Child with St John*, *c.* 1600
Oil on canvas (By Gracious Permission of H.M. the Queen)

A dramatic use of *chiaroscuro* is the dominant feature of this composition, no doubt an influence
from Caravaggio, a young contempory of the Carracci brothers. Annibale, regarded as the greatest
of the three brothers, spent many years working in Rome, although his studio was at the
Accademia in Bologna. His style is based on strict High Renaissance concepts: the study of Raphael
was all important in his work. This painting was bought in 1766 by Richard Dalton, the Royal
Surveyor and Keeper, and brought back to England for George III.

82. ABOVE Giovanni Battista Salvi (Sassoferrato), *The Madonna in Prayer*, before 1640
Oil on canvas (National Gallery, London)

A follower of Domenichino, Sassoferrato broke away from the High Baroque style and produced
several pictures of a simple, innocent nature. He has achieved an exceptional sweetness and purity in
the face of this Madonna.

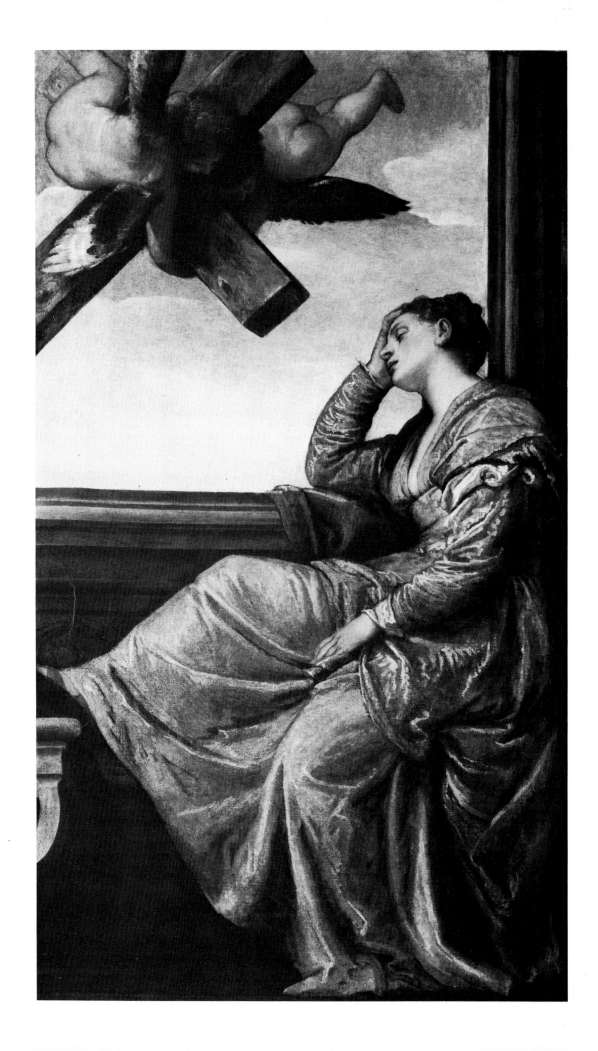

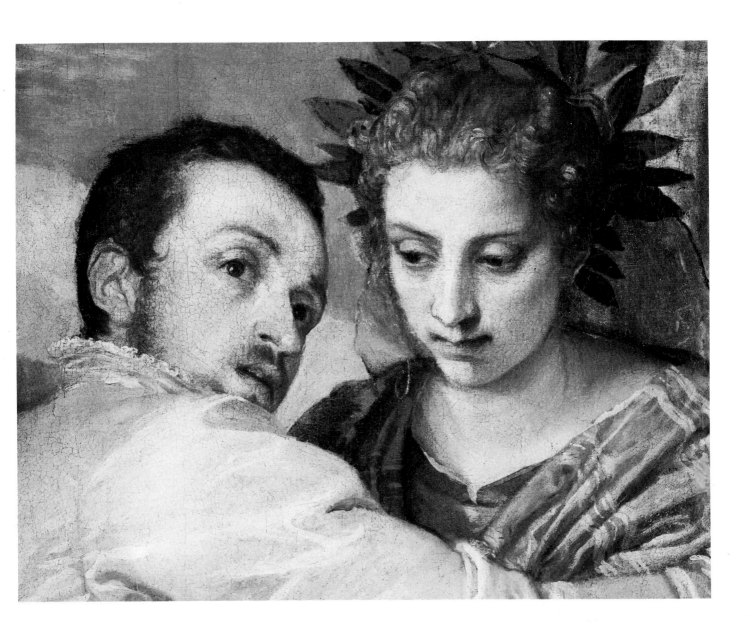

83. OPPOSITE Paolo Caliari (Veronese), *The Vision of St Helena*
Oil on canvas (National Gallery, London)

The Vision of St Helena is probably an early work, predating the vast biblical paintings which,
because of their worldly content, earned Veronese the Inquisitor's displeasure. Here Veronese shows
his superb mastery of the use of perspective in the strong diagonals of the composition and the almost
architectural pose of the sleeping St Helena.

84. ABOVE Paolo Caliari (Veronese), *Allegory of Vice and Virtue* (detail), *c.* 1580
Oil on canvas (Frick Collection, New York)

The story of Hercules meeting Vice and Virtue was a popular theme in Renaissance art and
literature. In Veronese's portrayal of this subject, Hercules is dressed in an elegant sixteenth-century
costume and is possibly an allegorized portrait of the artist.

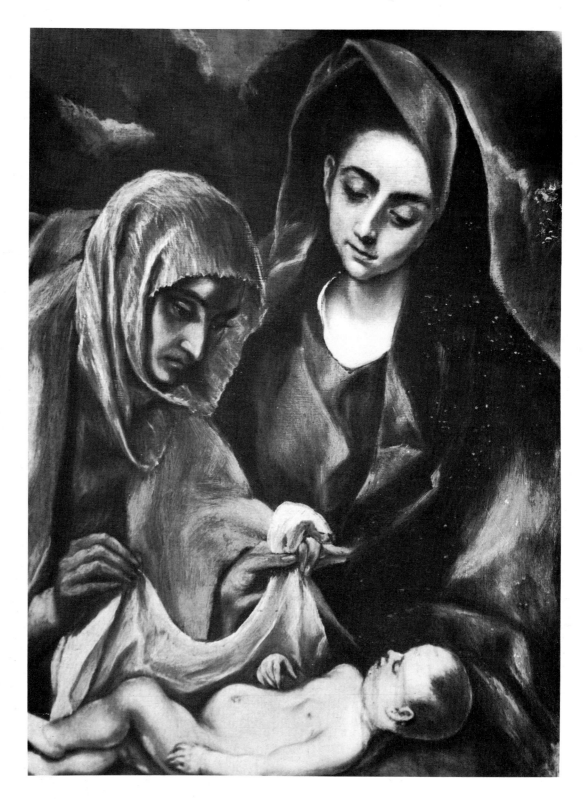

85. ABOVE Domenikos Theotocopoulos (El Greco), *Virgin and Child with St Anne*
Oil on canvas (St Vincente Museum, Toledo)

86. OPPOSITE Domenikos Theotocopoulos (El Greco), *Lady in a Fur Wrap*, 1577–8
Oil on canvas (Stirling Maxwell Collection, Pollock House, Glasgow)

These two paintings are excellent examples of El Greco's eclectic style. The *Virgin and Child with St Anne* has the strange elongation that is his hallmark, while the *Lady in a Fur Wrap* is far more detailed. In the first, he is concerned with emotion and religious feeling, whereas in the second he has clearly delighted in the delicate textures of fur, silk and skin. But the paintings are similar in their dramatic treatment of light and dark: in both, vivid patches of light are set against an inky background to heighten the importance of the subject.

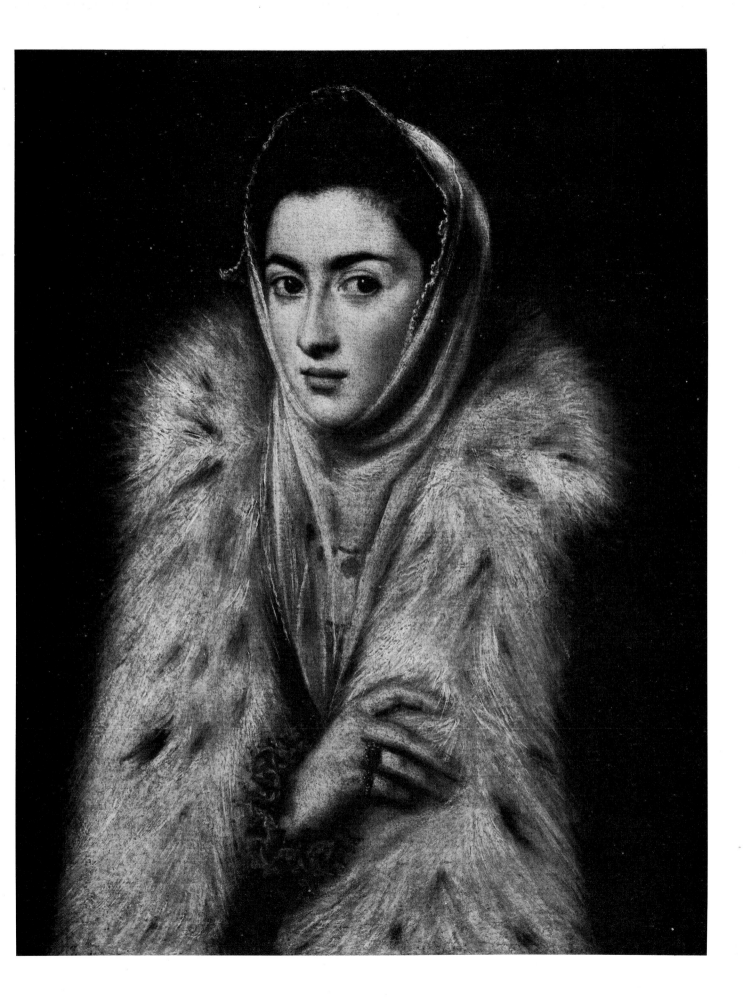

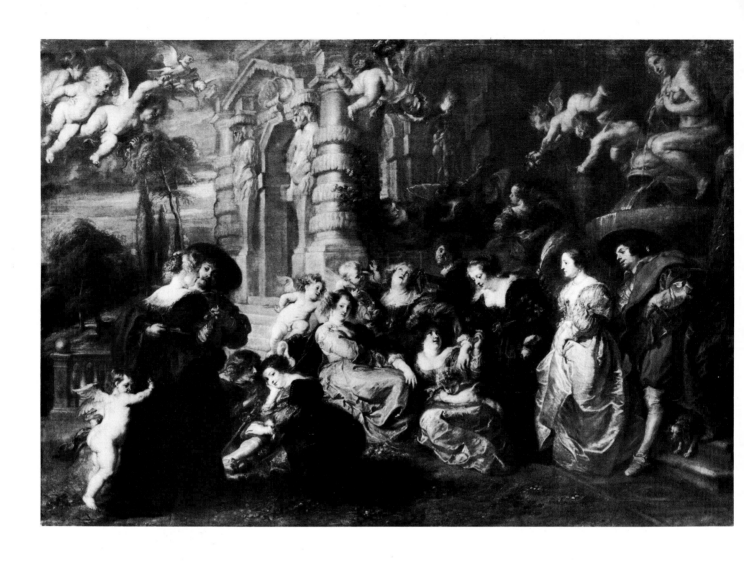

87. ABOVE Sir Peter Paul Rubens, *The Garden of Love*
Oil on panel (Prado, Madrid)

To the uninitiated, Rubens is often regarded as a painter of fat women: nothing could be more derogatory to the master of the art of design. His women are part of nature, innocent and abundant, and their weightiness is a feature of a carefully controlled scheme. Rubens has included himself as the cavalier on the left, and his young wife, Hélène Fourment, as the central figure below the pillar.

88. OPPOSITE Sir Peter Paul Rubens, *The Andromeda*
Oil on panel (Staatliche Museum, Berlin)

The Andromeda is an achievement of the highest technical skill. The soft luxuriance of flesh seems to absorb the glowing light and transmit its own: a dazzling feat, carried out with immense verve and confidence, and one that extremely few painters have ever equalled.

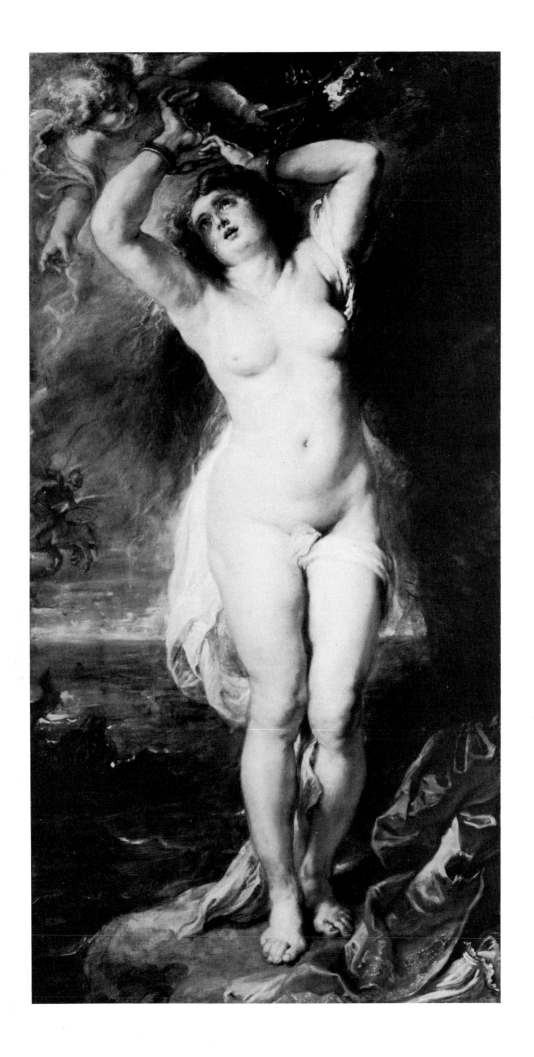

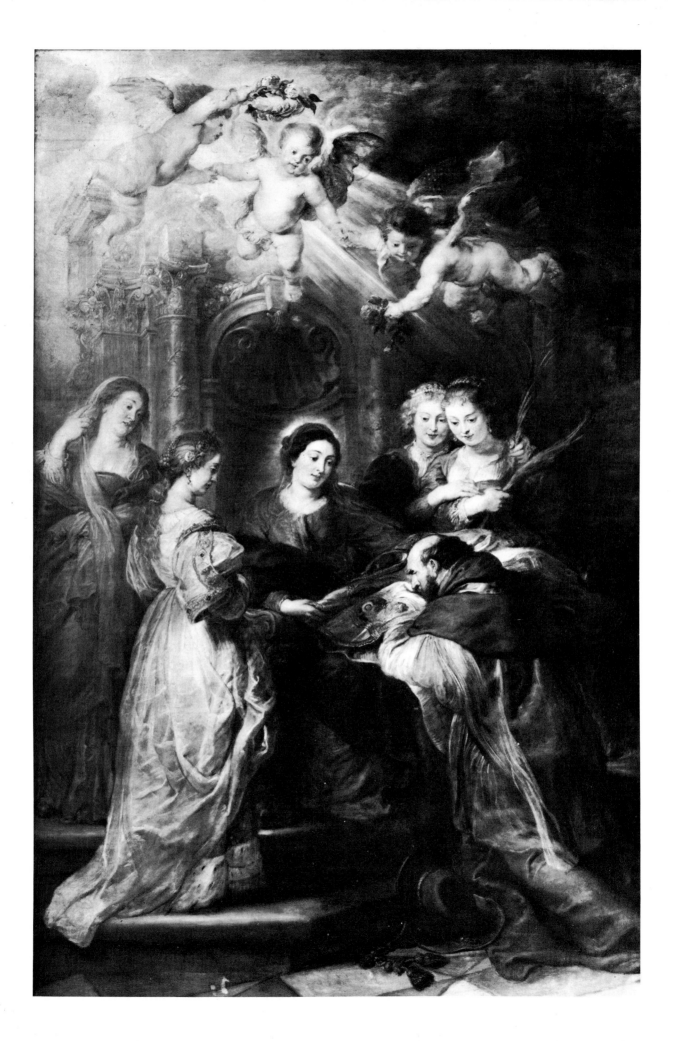

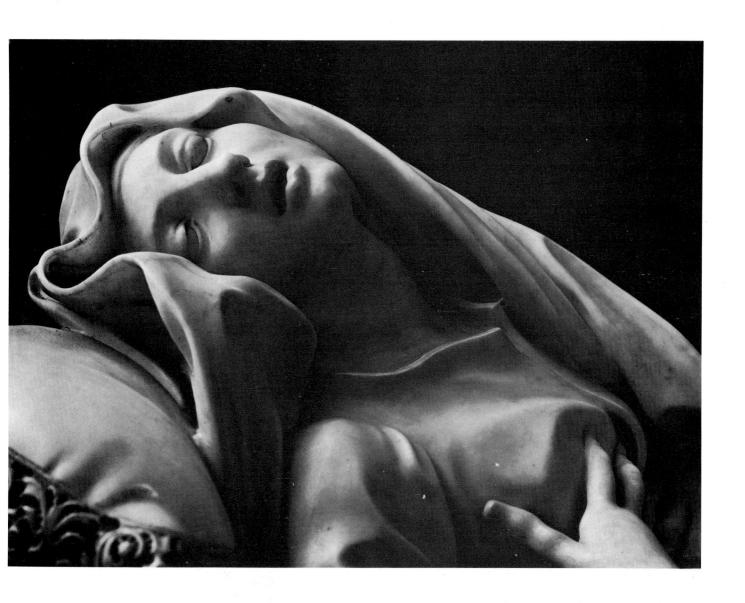

89. OPPOSITE Sir Peter Paul Rubens, *Ildefonso Triptych*, 1631–2
Oil on canvas (Kunsthistorisches Museum, Vienna)

Rubens, apart from being the master of the nude, was the greatest exponent of religious subjects of
his time. In this scene he depicts the vision of St Ildefonso, in which the Virgin, surrounded by
saints and angels, presents a heavenly robe to Ildefonso, and he kneels at her feet to receive it.

90. ABOVE Gianlorenzo Bernini, *The Blessed Ludovica Albertoni* (detail), 1671–4
Marble (Church of Francesco a Ripa, Rome)

Bernini was the dazzlingly precocious son of a late Mannerist sculptor who went to Rome *c.* 1605 to
work for Pope Paul V. The Pope's nephew, Cardinal Scipione Borghese, recognized the boy's
exceptional talent and became his patron. By his mid-twenties Bernini was hailed as the greatest
sculptor since Michelangelo. *The Blessed Ludovica Albertoni* is the lesser-known of two great works
in which he portrays saints in a state of divine ecstasy (the other is St Teresa), a theme which
allowed him to display his astonishing ability to express extreme emotion through the medium of
carved marble.

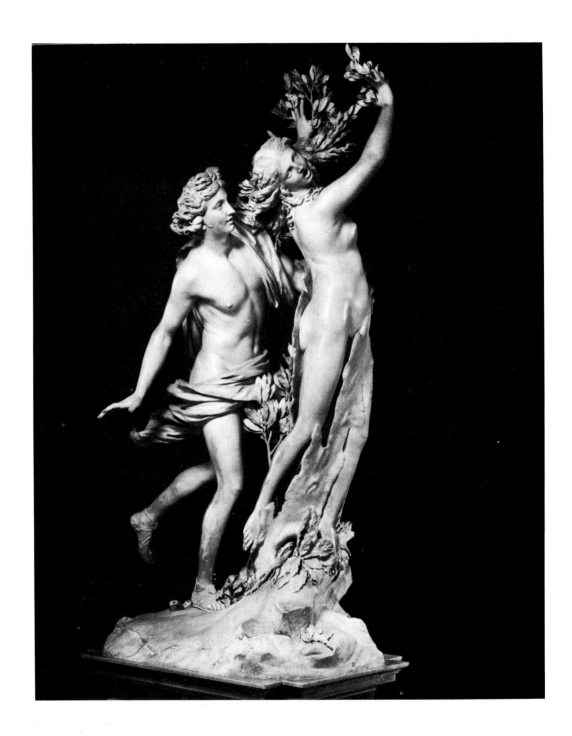

91. ABOVE Gianlorenzo Bernini, *Apollo and Daphne*, 1622–4
Marble (Borghese Gallery, Rome)

Cardinal Scipione Borghese commissioned this work when Bernini was only twenty-four. He was
already the perfect master of his medium: never had anyone made marble look so light and alive,
nor handled it with such fluidity as to convey the awful speed of Daphne's transformation from
woman to tree.

92. OPPOSITE Paolo Caliari (Veronese), *Portrait of a Woman (La Belle Nani)*
Oil on canvas (Louvre, Paris)

Veronese was patronized by the patrician families of Venice, and in his *Portrait of a Woman* he shows
the rich opulence of the reigning beauties of the time. A splendid dress, adorned with lace and
jewels, and fashionable pearl-drop ear-rings, enhance the sensuality of her ample, voluptuous
shoulders, full lips and indolent eyes.

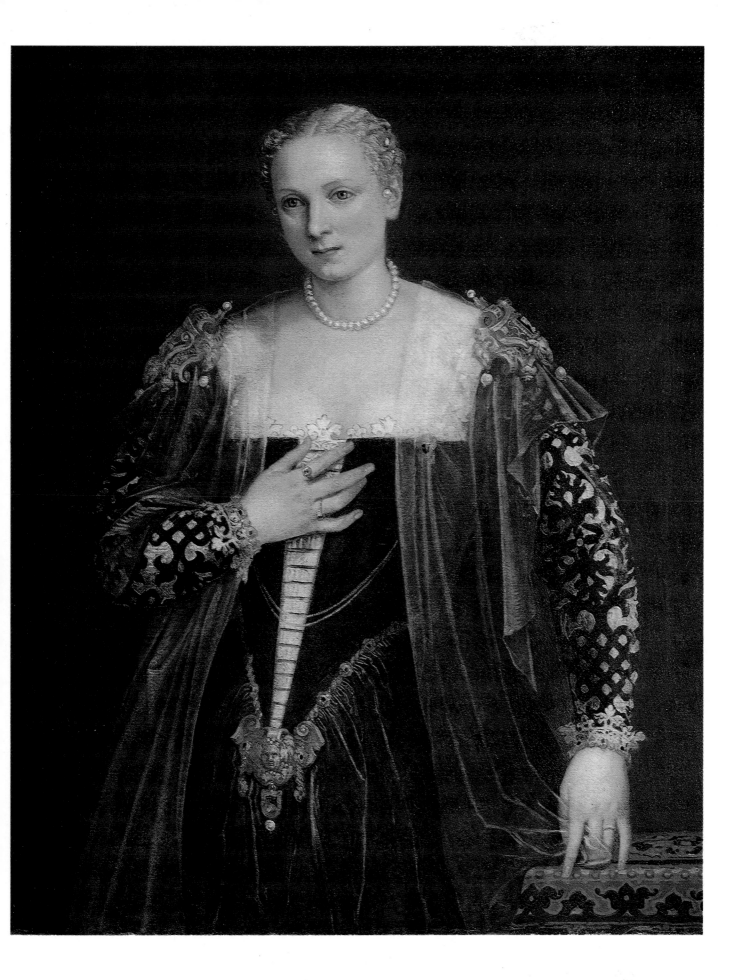

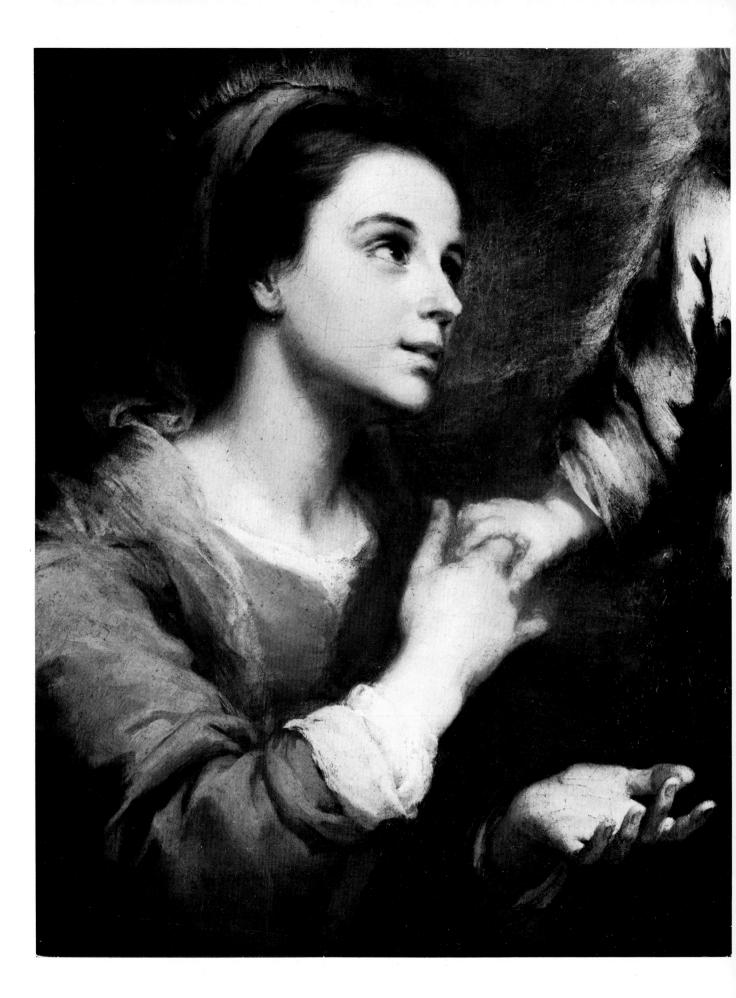

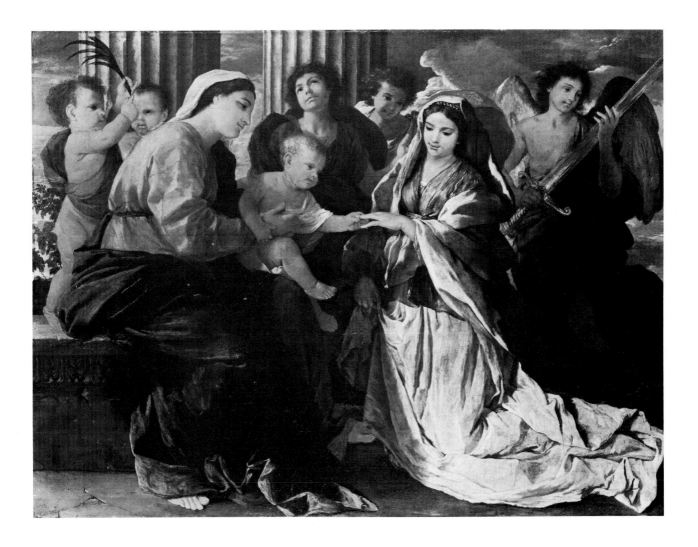

93. ABOVE Bartolomé Esteban Murillo, *The Two Trinities* (detail), *c.* 1681–2
Oil on canvas (National Gallery, London)

Murillo lived most of his life in Seville, where he founded and was the first President of the Seville
Academy. His undemanding devotional pictures enjoyed immense popularity in Spain well into
the nineteenth century. They are characterized by their tender piety, often bordering on
sentimentality, but his delicate colouring and free brush strokes give them an appealing humanity
and warmth.

94. OPPOSITE Nicolas Poussin, *Sacra Conversazione*
Oil on canvas (National Gallery of Scotland, Edinburgh)

Poussin, though French by birth, spent most of his working life in Rome. The *Sacra Conversazione*
displays two important influences in his work: the fluted columns and carved palmette frieze on the
stone seat firmly place the scene in Antiquity, while the figure of St Anne shows the influence of
Raphael. The undulating rhythm of the figures and the use of strongly contrasted light and dark
areas demonstrates, however, that Poussin had also assimilated and contributed to the
contemporary Baroque style.

95. OVERLEAF Guido Reni, *Venus and Cupid*, 1626
Oil on canvas (Toledo Museum, Ohio)

Venus is shown playing with her son, Cupid, and surrounded by her traditional attributes: red roses
and cooing doves. By the subtlety of his lighting, Guido has created a statuesque ideal of feminine
beauty. His figures, classical in origin, form a graceful and flowing composition. According to
Guido's biographer, Malvasia, this Venus was painted for a goldsmith in exchange for a diamond.
Because of this, the painting was known for a long time as *Il Diamante*, a title it richly deserves.

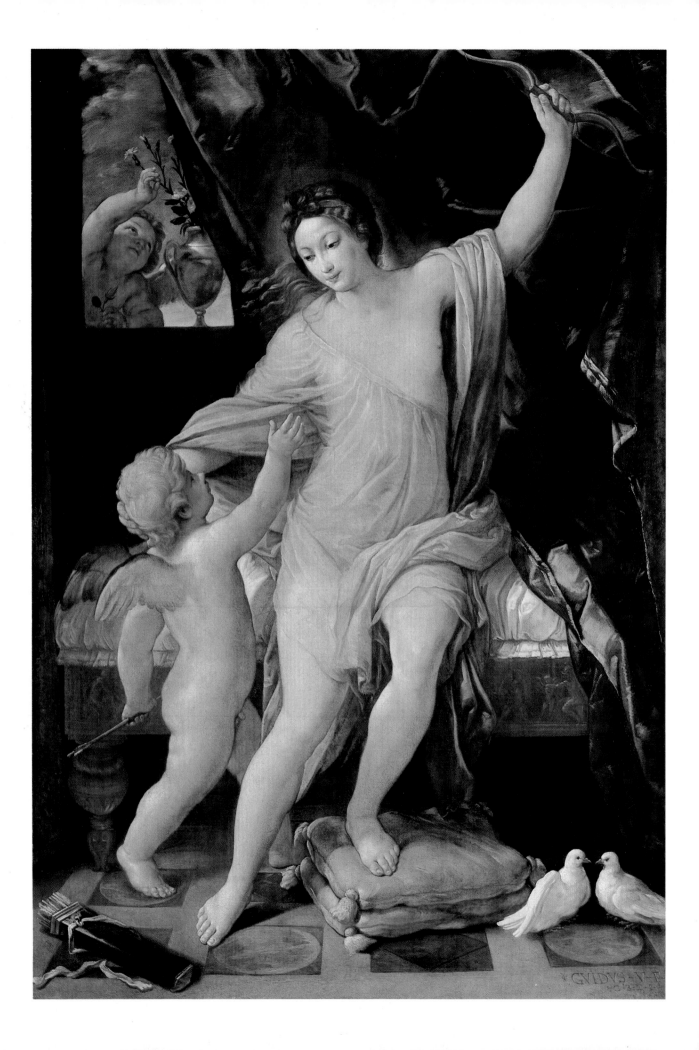

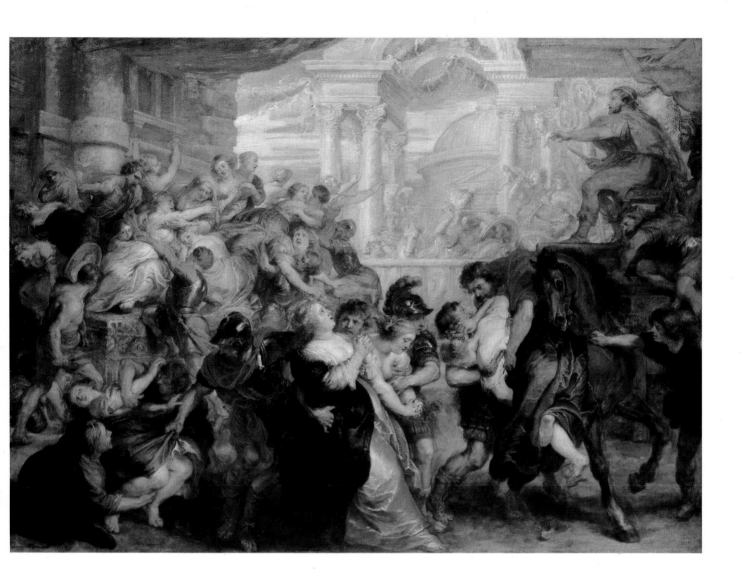

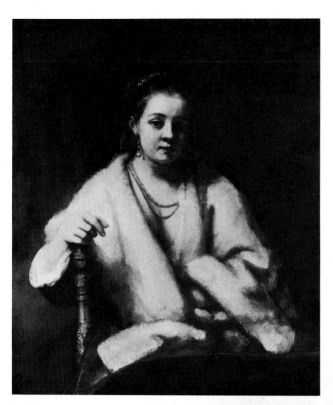
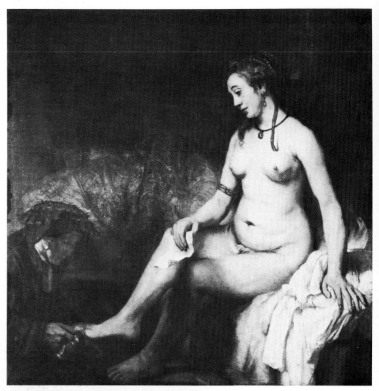

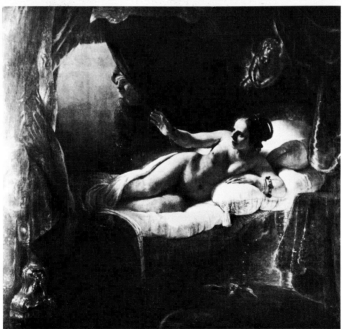

96. PRECEDING PAGE Sir Peter Paul Rubens, *The Rape of the Sabines*, 1635
Oil on panel (National Gallery, London)

This mass of twisting, turning bodies, brilliantly contained within the picture, is a pure expression
of Rubens' High Baroque style. The textures of flesh, draperies, helmets, plumes and marble have a
tangible reality which combines magnificently with the elements of movement and colour.

97. TOP LEFT Rembrandt van Rijn, *Hendrickje Stoffels*, 1659
Oil on canvas (National Gallery, London)

Hendrickje Stoffels is the sitter in many of Rembrandt's later works. A few years after his wife
Saskia died in 1642, Hendrickje became his mistress, and although she bore him a daughter, they
never married. This was probably due to the strict conditions of Saskia's will: had Rembrandt
remarried, the income from the will would have been stopped.

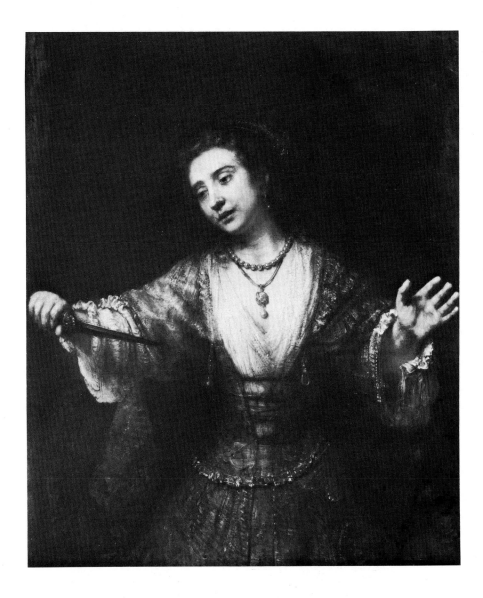

100. ABOVE Rembrandt van Rijn, *Lucretia*, 1664
Oil on canvas (National Gallery of Art, Washington DC: Andrew W. Mellon Collection)

98. OPPOSITE ABOVE RIGHT Rembrandt van Rijn, *Bathsheba*, 1654
Oil on canvas (Louvre, Paris)

Bathsheba, probably modelled by Hendrickje, is entirely unclassical in style, though the
composition derives from antique reliefs. The beauty of her thoughtful, intelligent gaze is very
different in its character from the coolness and vacancy of the Renaissance ideal.

99. OPPOSITE BELOW Rembrandt van Rijn, *Danae*, 1636
Oil on canvas (Hermitage, Leningrad)

The body of Danae, lit by celestial light, most closely represents Rembrandt's ideal of beauty; even
so, she is by no means a conventional or classical ideal. The undulating curves of her body, repeated
in the plump pillow and mattress, are a wonderful contrast to the rich material and gilded furniture
in the room. Her outstretched hand is the key to the composition, as it not only defines the
perspective but also indicates the presence of Zeus as the source of light.

100. ABOVE Rembrandt van Rijn, *Lucretia*, 1664
Oil on canvas (National Gallery of Art, Washington DC: Andrew W. Mellon Collection)

101. OVERLEAF Rembrandt van Rijn, *Lucretia*, 1666
Oil on canvas (Institute of Arts, Minneapolis)

The theme of Lucretia at the moment of her suicide strongly attracted Rembrandt as it combined
the main elements to which he inclined in his later work: drama, tension and emotion. The figure
of Lucretia was based yet again on Hendrickje.

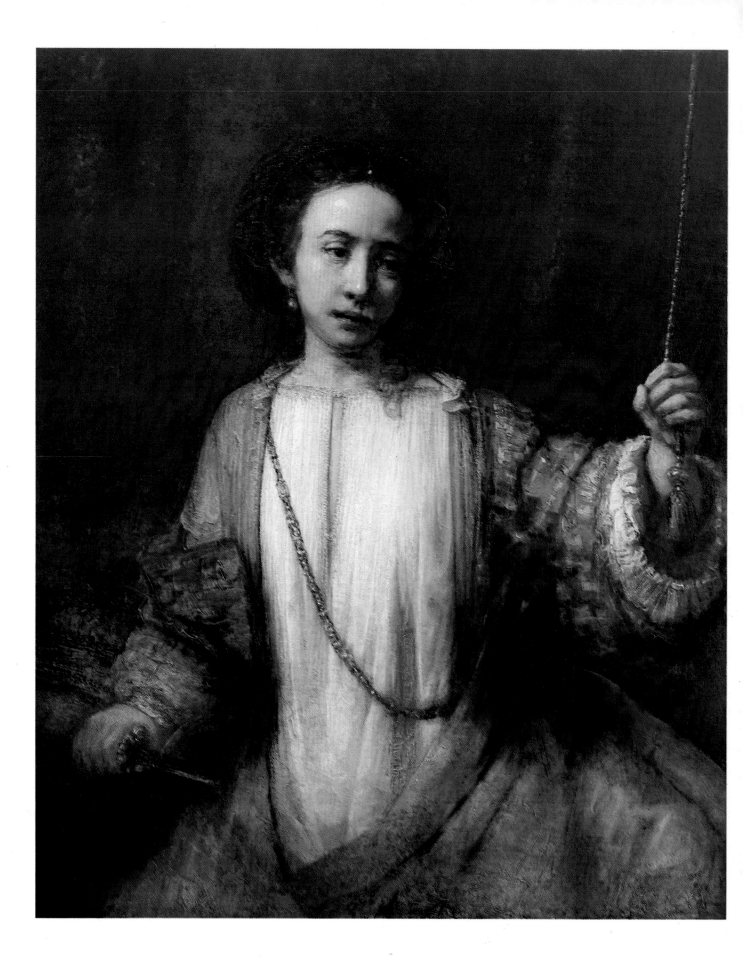

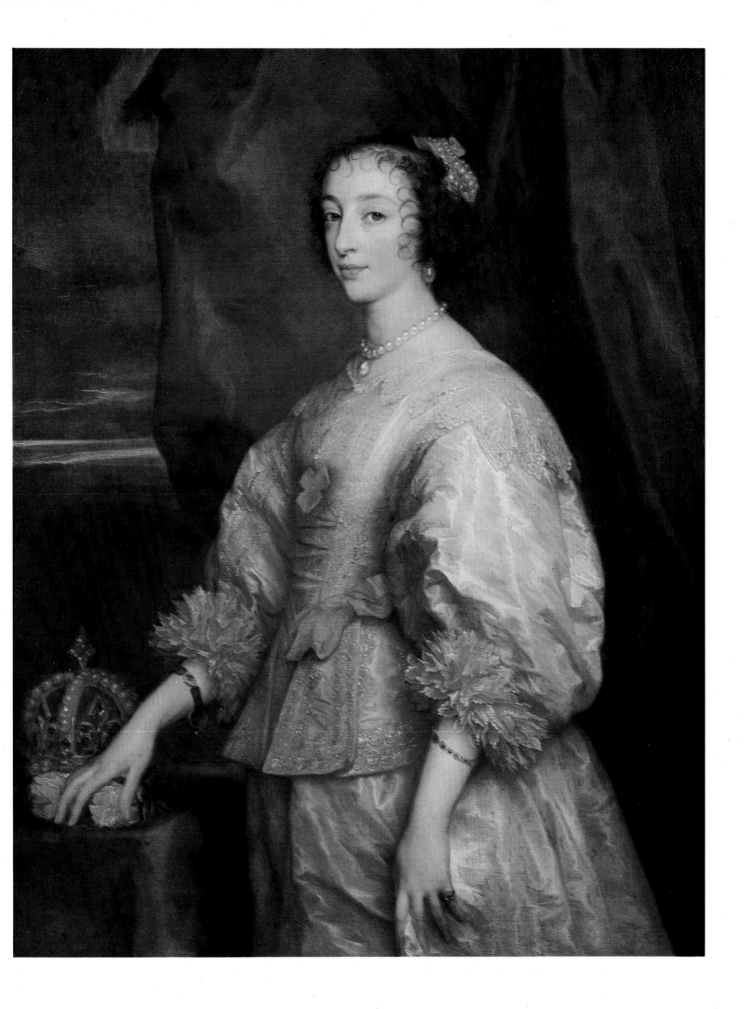

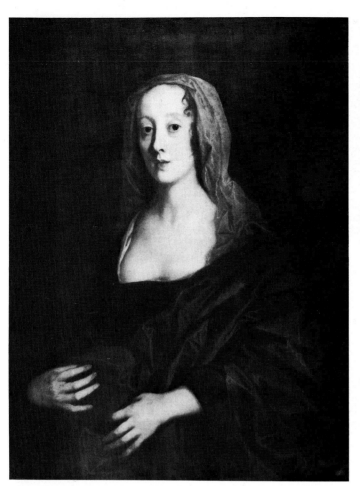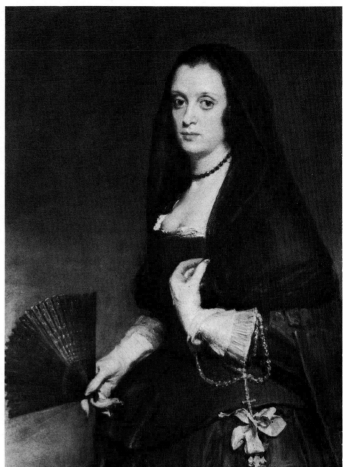

102. PRECEDING PAGE Sir Anthony Van Dyck, *Queen Henrietta Maria*, *c*. 1632
Oil on canvas (By Gracious Permission of H.M. the Queen)

Henrietta Maria, wife of Charles I, was an acknowledged beauty. Her exquisite colouring and fine features, combined with the opulence of her clothes and jewels, made her the perfect model for Van Dyck, who made many portraits of her.

103. ABOVE LEFT Sir Peter Lely, *Portrait of a Lady*, *c*. 1647
Oil on canvas (Aberconway Collection)

This strong and compelling portrait has a simplicity and unadorned directness remarkable in a painting by Lely, who, with his large studio, dominated fashionable Restoration portraiture.

104. ABOVE RIGHT Diego Velazquez, *The Lady with a Fan*
Oil on canvas (Wallace Collection, London)

In the Autumn of 1623 Velazquez was appointed Court Painter to Philip IV of Spain, and was promised that he alone would paint portraits of the new King. *The Lady with a Fan* is one of the very few pictures Velazquez painted of a woman outside the Spanish court circle, and it is perhaps this, and the fact that there are two other paintings of her, that has led to the suggestion that she may have been his wife.

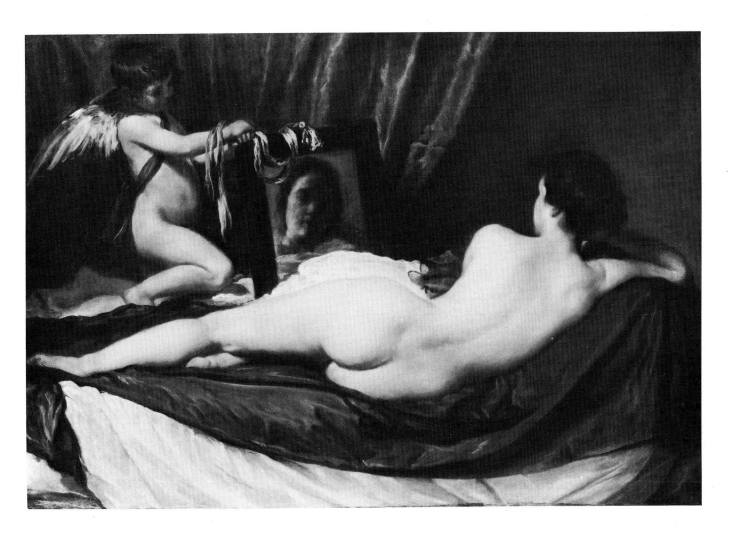

105. ABOVE Diego Velazquez, *The Toilet of Venus (The Rokeby Venus)*, 1648–9
Oil on canvas (National Gallery, London)

Although Velazquez is known to have painted at least four pictures of female nudes, a subject extremely rare in Spanish seventeenth-century painting, this is the only one to have survived. It may have been painted shortly before or during the artist's second visit to Italy in 1649–51, and it shows strongly the influence on Velazquez of the great sixteenth-century Venetian painters, especially Titian. The painting, which takes its name from a previous owner, John Morritt of Rokeby Park in Yorkshire, was badly slashed in 1914 by a suffragette, but has since been restored.

106. OVERLEAF LEFT Giovanni Battista (Giambattista) Tiepolo, *An Allegory of Venus with Time, c.* 1754
Oil on canvas (National Gallery, London)

Tiepolo, the greatest decorative artist of the eighteenth-century, painted this allegory in the 1750s, when he was at the height of his fame. It was originally part of a ceiling decoration in a Venetian palace of the Contarini family, and may have been commissioned to celebrate the birth of an heir. This would explain the subject matter and the title 'The Confinement of Venus' which Giovanni Domenico Tiepolo gave to the etching he made after his father's painting.

107. OVERLEAF RIGHT Jean Honoré Fragonard, *The Lover Crowned, c.* 1772
Oil on canvas (Frick Collection, New York)

This is the third of the original four panels of the series *The Progress of Love*, commissioned by Madame du Barry for the new dining pavilion of her château at Louveciennes. Although they are now regarded as outstanding examples of French eighteenth-century decorative art, Madame du Barry rejected them, and Fragonard kept them until 1790. After adding two more large panels and eight small ones, he installed the whole series in the salon of his cousin's house.

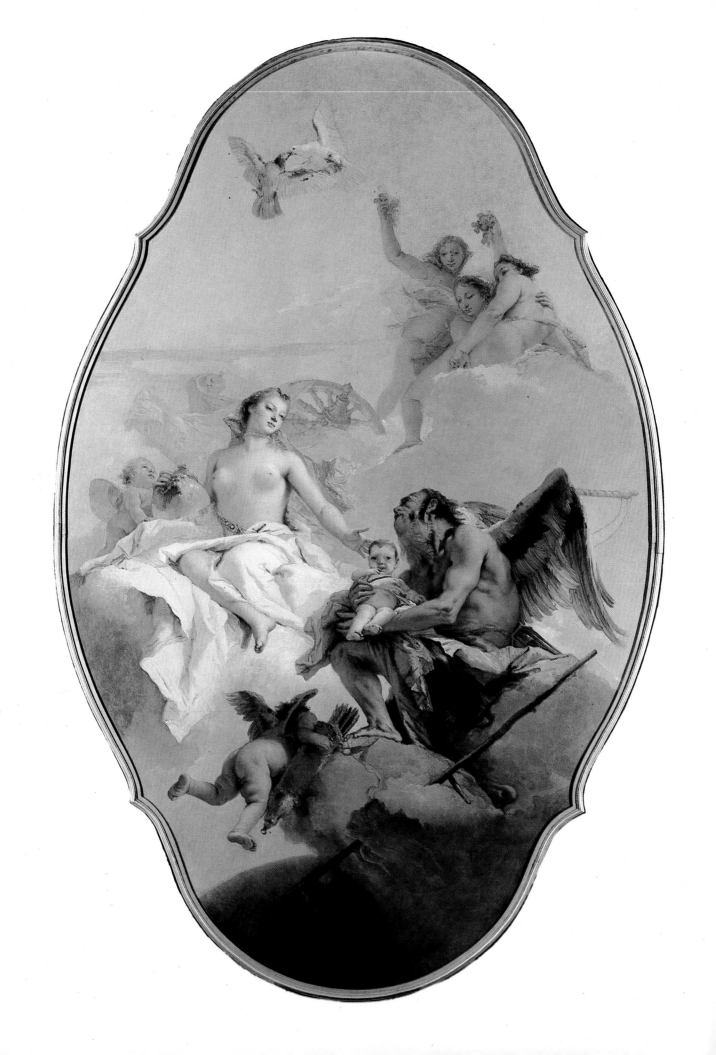

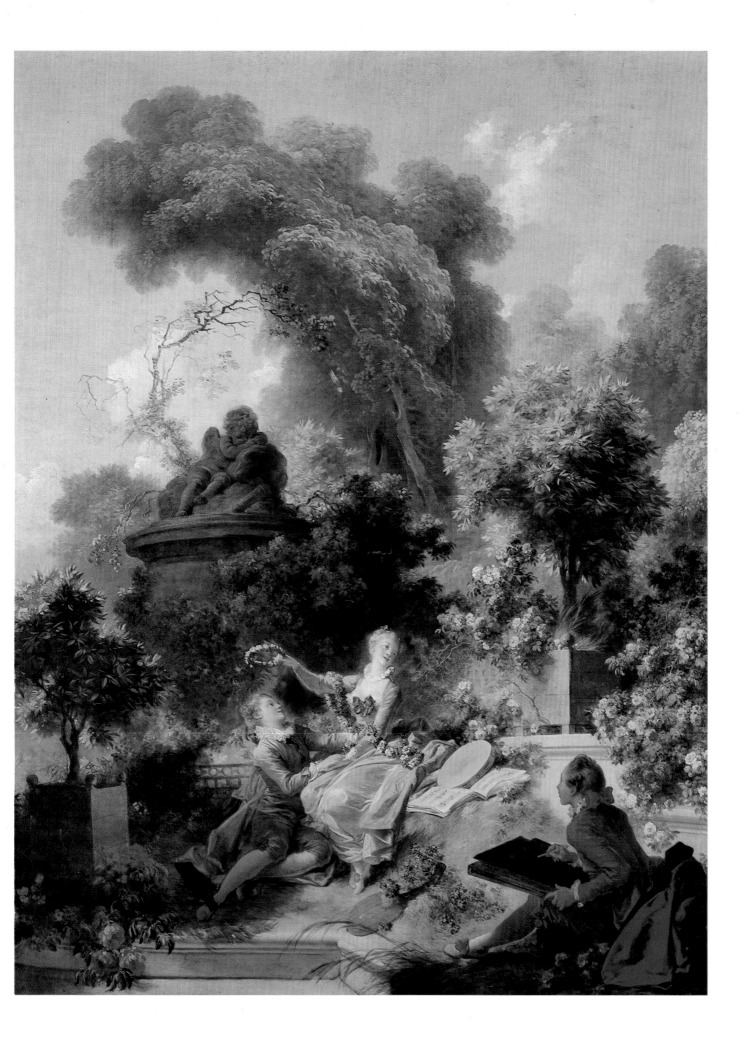

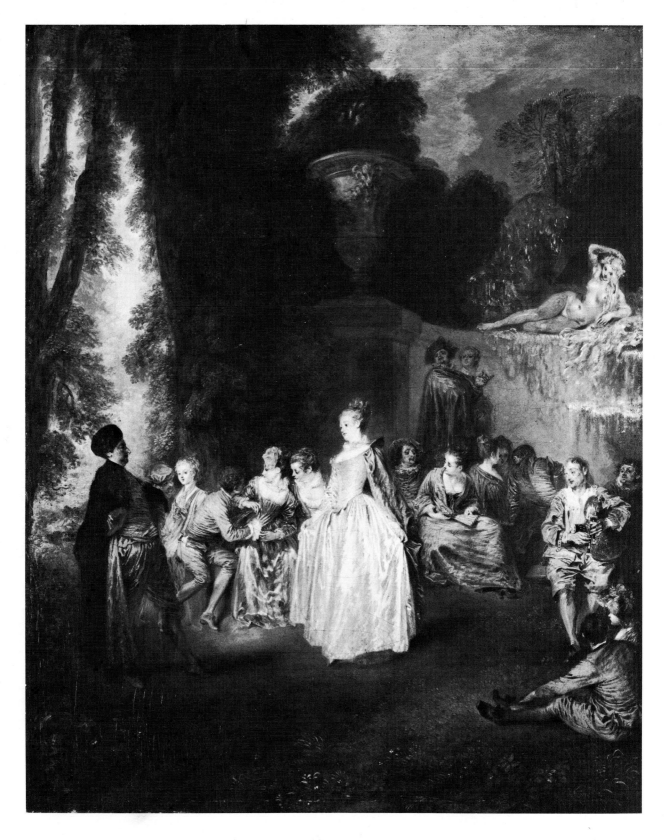

108. Antoine Watteau, *Fêtes Venetiennes, c.* 1717
Oil on canvas (National Gallery of Scotland, Edinburgh)

This painting possibly takes its title from *Les Festes Venetiennes*, a ballet by Danchet and Campra
performed in Paris from 1710 onwards. It is a fine example of the many charming paintings of
idyllic outdoor music parties that earned Voltaire's rather damning (and now challenged)
comment: 'Watteau was quite successful with the little figures that he drew and grouped well; but
he never did anything great; he was incapable of it' (*Le Temple du Gout*, 1731). Watteau has
included himself in this painting as the bagpipe player on the far right of the group.

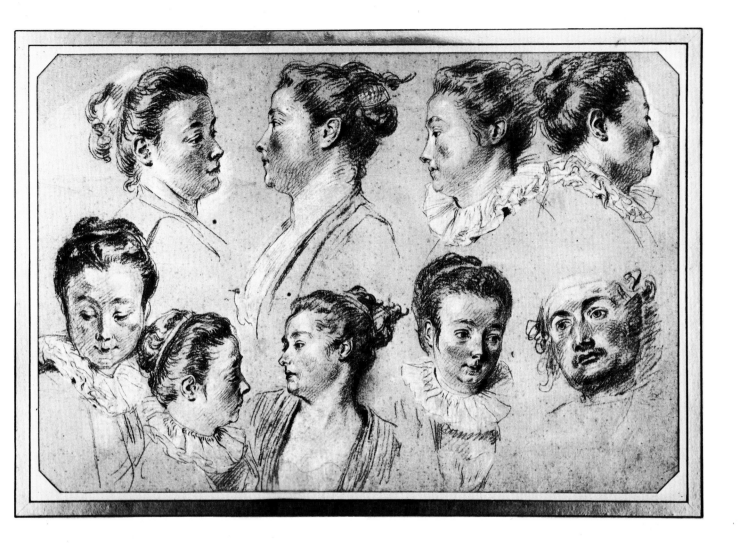

109. ABOVE Antoine Watteau, *Sheet of Studies*
Black, red and white crayon (Louvre, Paris)

Watteau made hundreds of superb drawings – studies of heads, figures, hands and draperies in coloured crayon – which he kept in bound volumes and referred to when starting a painting, gathering together whatever components he needed. These sheets of studies are some of his loveliest work.

110. OVERLEAF LEFT Thomas Gainsborough, *Mary, Countess Howe, c.* 1765
Oil on canvas (The Iveagh Bequest, Kenwood House, London)

Between 1760 and 1774 Gainsborough lived and worked in Bath, and it was during this period that he painted some of his most elegant portraits. He studied the old masters, particularly Van Dyck, whose influence can be seen in the exquisite painting of the Countess's silk and lace dress, its sophistication an effective contrast to the rustic landscape setting.

111. OVERLEAF RIGHT Allan Ramsay, *The Painter's Wife, c.* 1755
Oil on canvas (National Gallery of Scotland, Edinburgh)

Ramsay, a Scotsman, received his formative training in Rome and Naples. On returning to England in 1738 he settled in London and was immediately successful as a portrait painter. In the early 1750s he wrote two essays, 'On Ridicule' and 'On Taste', which commend naturalism in art. In this superb portrait of his second wife he combines the elegance and skill he learnt in Rome with the naturalism he preached in London.

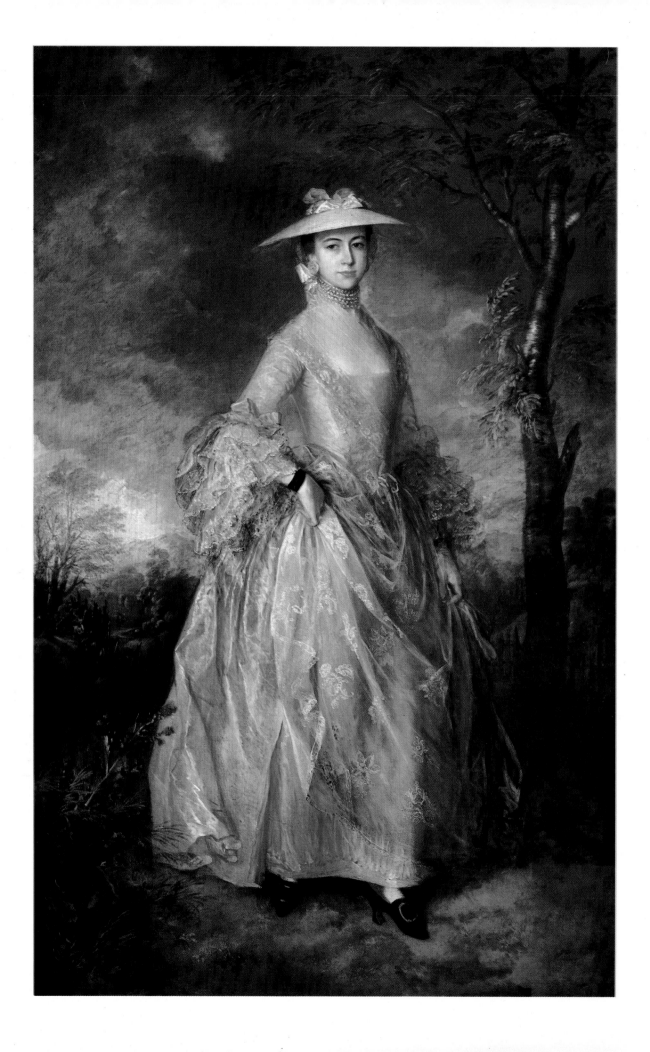

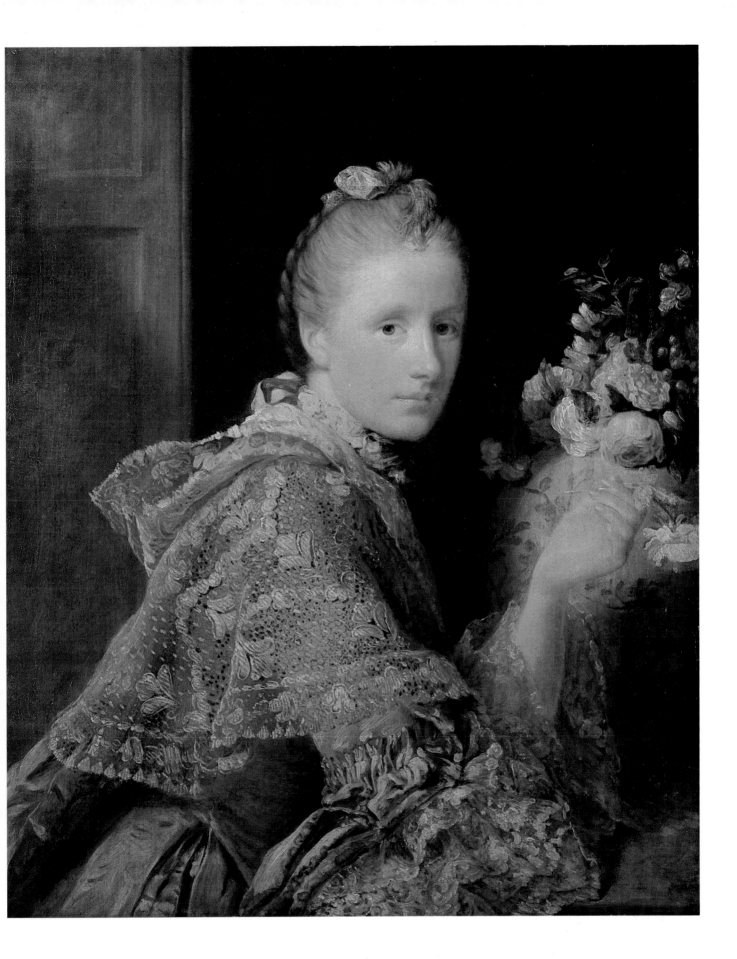

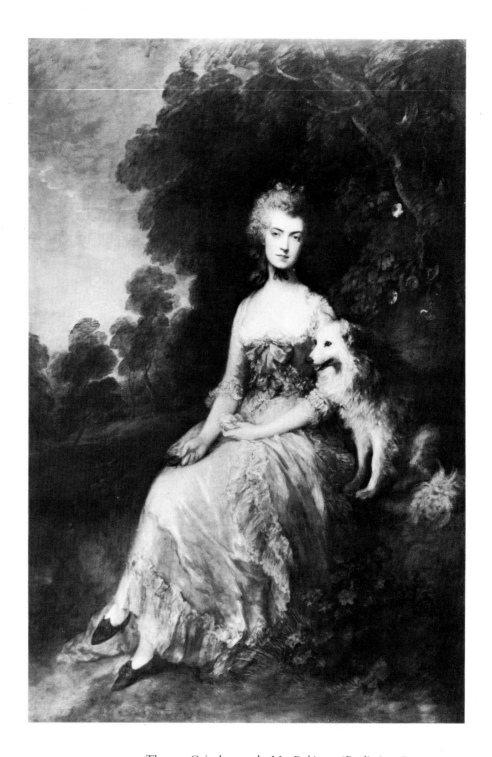

112. ABOVE Thomas Gainsborough, *Mrs Robinson (Perdita)*, 1781
Oil on canvas (Wallace Collection, London)

Mary Robinson, an actress, attracted the attention of the Prince of Wales when she appeared as
Perdita in 1779. She became his mistress, and it was he who commissioned this portrait and the
miniature of him that she holds in her hand: a bill from Gainsborough to the Prince of Wales, dated
June 1784, includes the item 'a full length of Mrs Robinson £105.0'.

113. OPPOSITE John Hoppner, *Mrs Henry Richmond Gale*, c. 1781
Oil on canvas (Toledo Museum, Ohio: Gift of Edward Drummond Libbey)

John Hoppner, the son of a German surgeon who attended George III, spent his boyhood as a
chorister at St James's Palace before being sent by the King to the Royal Academy in 1775. He
became extremely popular as a portraitist, and was made Portrait Painter to the Prince of Wales in
1793. This is a particularly spirited example of his work, in which he has taken full advantage of the
striking bone structure of the sitter.

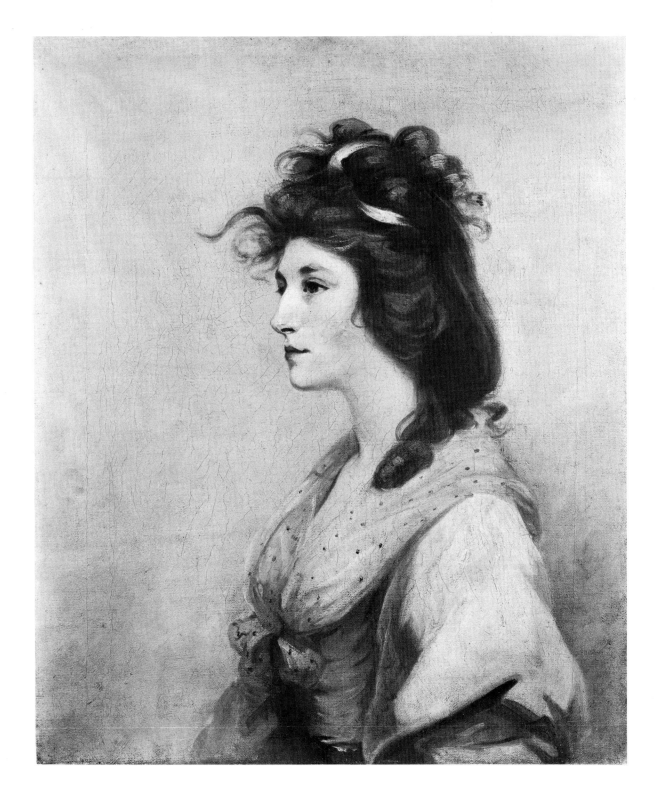

114. OVERLEAF LEFT George Romney, *Lady Hamilton as Circe*, c. 1782
Oil on canvas (Tate Gallery, London)

Romney met the ravishingly beautiful Emma Hamilton in 1781 and became obsessed with her. He painted her over and over again, often casting her in an historical or, as here, mythological role as Circe, the enchantress.

115. OVERLEAF RIGHT Francisco Goya, *Maja Desnuda*, c. 1798–1800
Oil on canvas (Prado, Madrid)

The most famous *maja* of Goya's time was the aristocratic but highly unconventional thirteenth Duchess of Alba, whom Goya painted several times. The speculation that she posed for this blatantly erotic and exquisite painting understandably caused a furore in Spanish society.

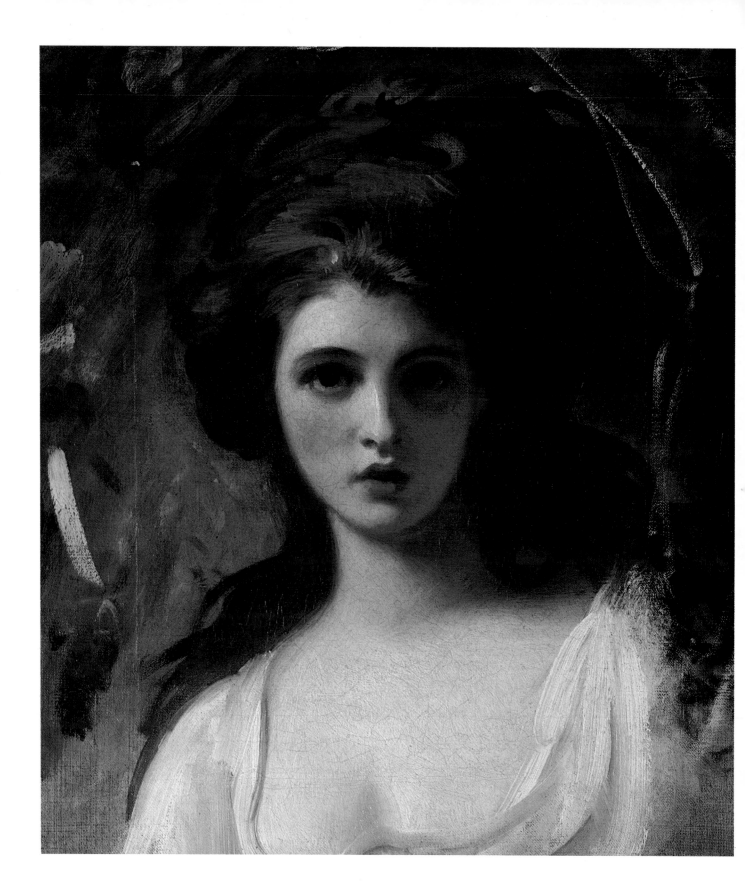

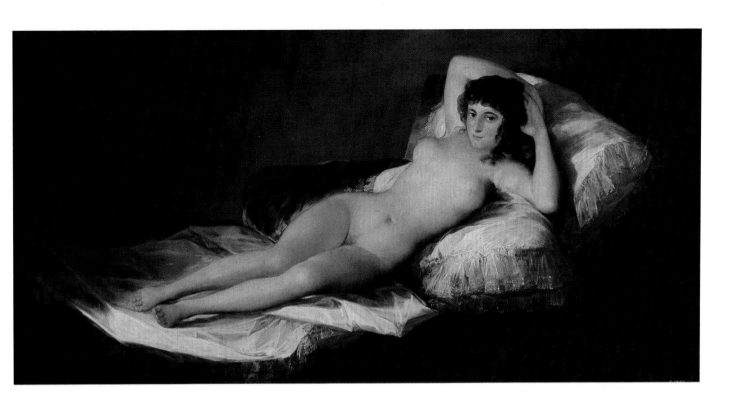

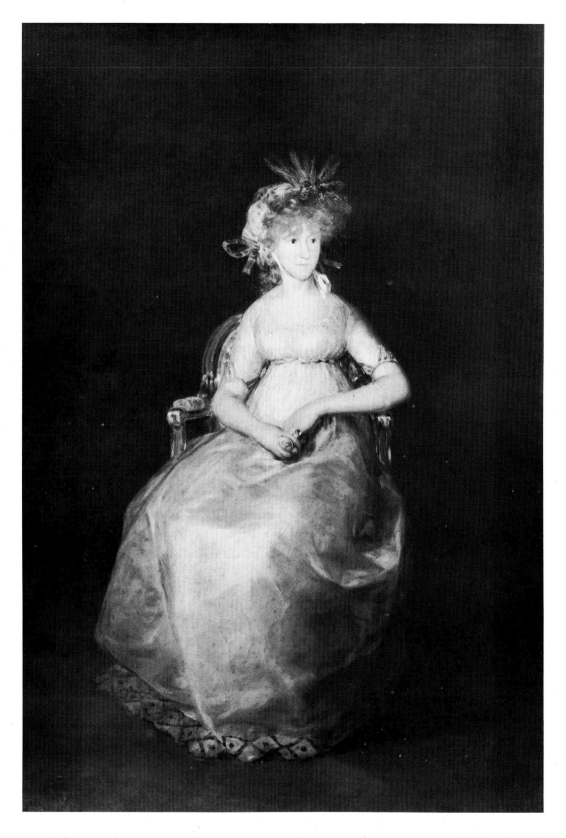

116. Francisco Goya, *Condesa de Chinchon*, 1800
Oil on canvas (Duke of Sueca Collection, Madrid)

The Condesa de Chinchon was the illegitimate daughter of the Infante D. Luis and a lady of Aragon, Doña Maria Teresa de Vallabriga. First painted by Goya in 1783 when she was six years old, she married Don Manuel Godoy, Duke of Alcudia and of Sueca, Minister of Charles IV. An extract from a letter from Queen Maria Luisa to Godoy, '. . . we hope she will go on well until all is over', and the style of the Condesa's dress, both suggest that this portrait was painted when she was expecting a child.

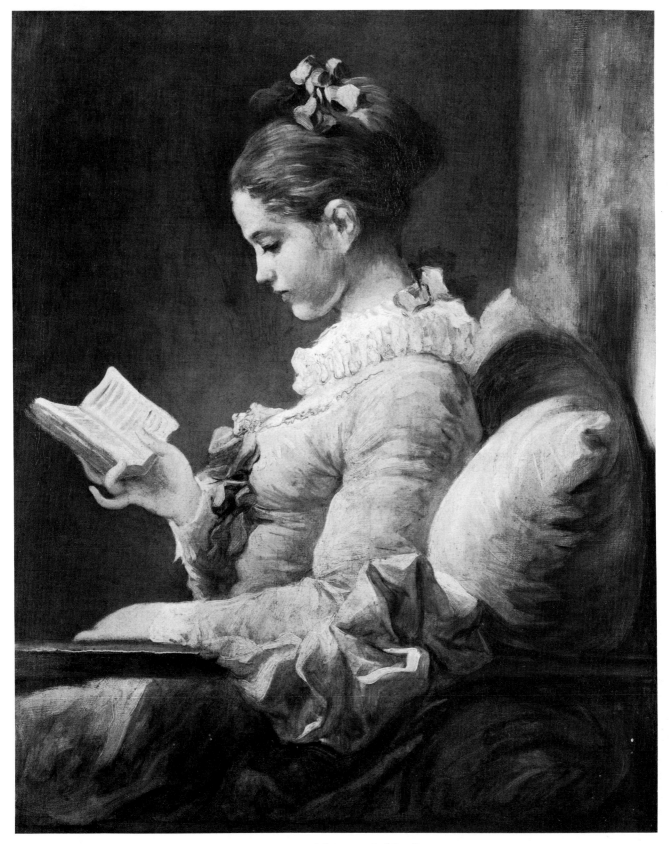

117. Jean Honoré Fragonard, *Young Girl Reading*, c. 1775
Oil on canvas (National Gallery of Art, Washington DC: Jules S. Bache Collection)

No painter epitomizes an era more precisely than does Fragonard the age of pre-revolutionary, eighteenth-century France. The prettiness of the woman he painted and the sumptuousness of their clothes so well suited the hedonism of the reigns of Louis XV and Louis XVI that, in the eyes of the revolutionaries, he was equated with it. He died, forgotten, unfashionable and in extreme poverty in Paris in 1806.

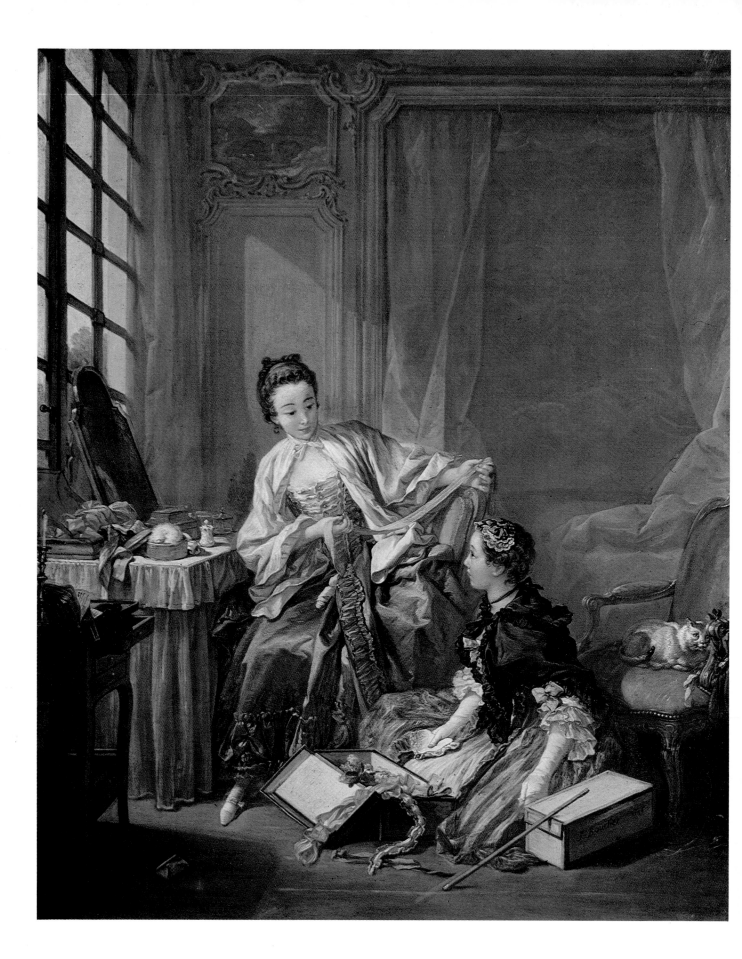

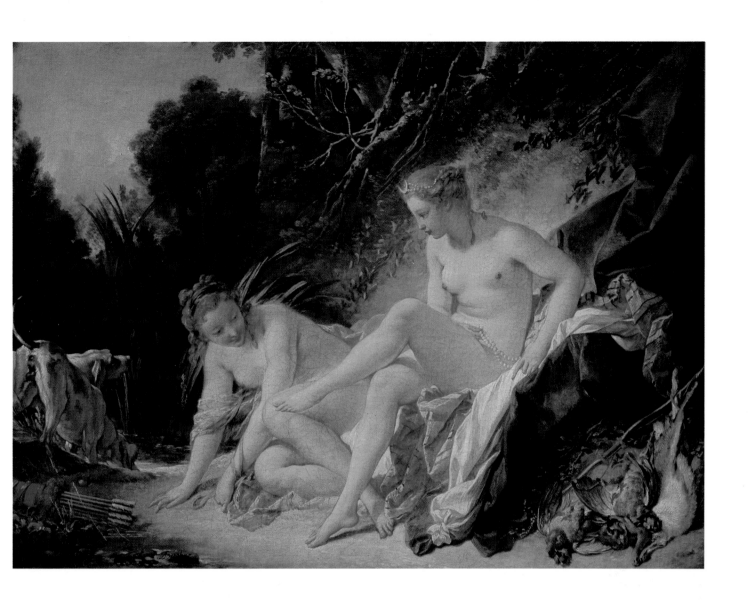

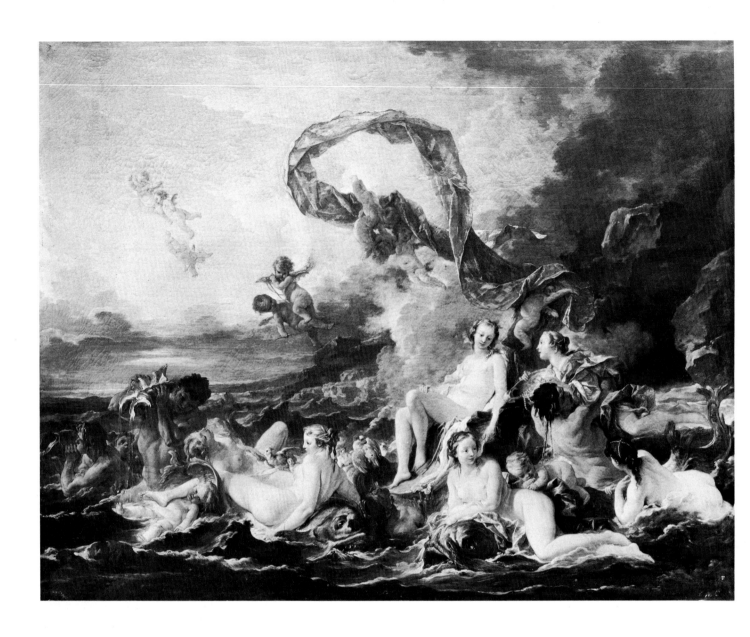

118. PRECEDING PAGES LEFT François Boucher, *The Milliner*, 1746
Oil on canvas (Nationalmuseum, Stockholm)

119. PRECEDING PAGES RIGHT François Boucher, *Diana Resting after her Bath*, 1742
Oil on canvas (Louvre, Paris)

Boucher was the friend and protégé of Madame de Pompadour, and his paintings reflect the luxury and prettiness of her time. In *The Milliner* he has taken obvious delight in painting the fashionable decoration of the room as well as the equally stylish central figure. However, in *Diana Resting after Her Bath*, the Arcadian landscape is entirely subordinate to the voluptuous perfection of the two nudes. Renoir described this painting as 'a work I have adored all my life, like a first love . . . Boucher was an artist who really mastered the art of portraying the female body'.

120. ABOVE François Boucher, *The Triumph of Amphitrite*, 1740
Oil on canvas (Nationalmuseum, Stockholm)

In *The Triumph of Amphitrite*, a riot of glowing, naked flesh, Boucher has concentrated the essence of his imaginary world, filling his canvas with beautiful, langorous goddesses, and with nymphs, maenads and cherubs. Everything, from the clouds to the dolphins is curved and soft, typifying the happy, light harmony of the Rococo style.

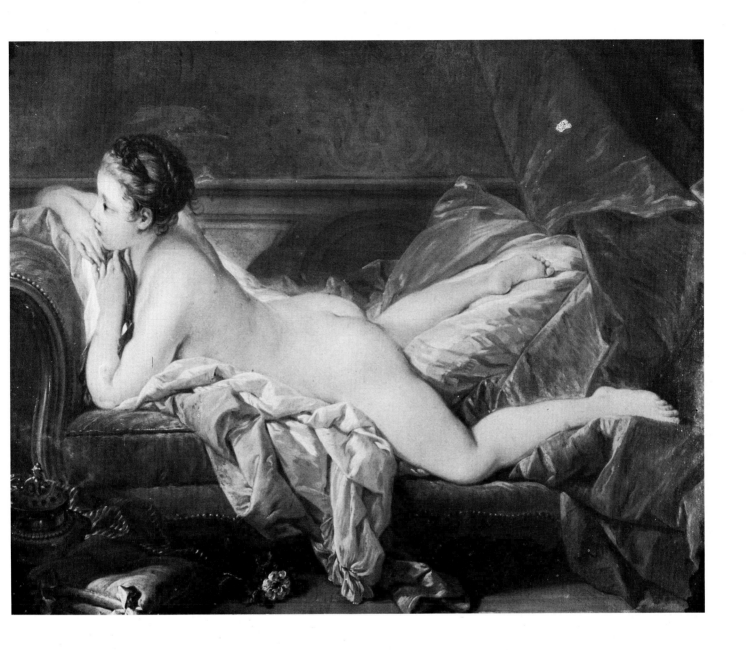

121. ABOVE François Boucher, *Louise O'Murphy*, 1752
Oil on canvas (Alte Pinakothek, Munich)

Louise O'Murphy was an Irish girl whose father, a shoemaker, followed King James II to France
and settled in Rouen. Her three sisters became Parisian courtesans, and in their company she met
Casanova, who was so enchanted by her that he arranged for Boucher to paint her in the nude. It
was through Boucher that she came to the notice of Louis XV; she became one of the King's many
mistresses and had two children by him.

122. OVERLEAF ABOVE LEFT Jacques-Louis David, *Madame Récamier*, 1800
Oil on canvas (Louvre, Paris)

123. OVERLEAF FAR RIGHT Antonio Canova, *Paolina Borghese*, 1808
Marble (Borghese Gallery, Rome)

Madame Récamier, the loveliest and most elegant woman of her time, was the perfect model for
David. She dressed in simple, loose robes of white muslin, and decorated her house with
Neo-Classical furniture. She was the declared enemy of Napoleon, whose sister, Paolina Borghese,
was portrayed eight years later in a similar pose, but virtually naked, as Venus, by the celebrated
sculptor Canova.

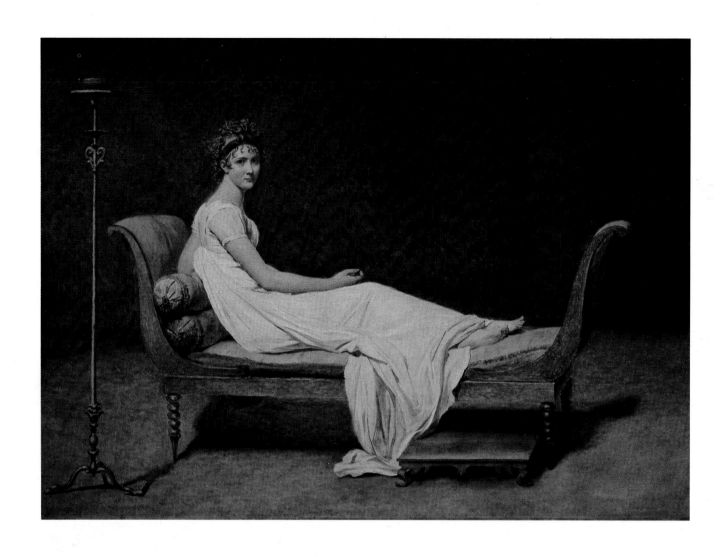

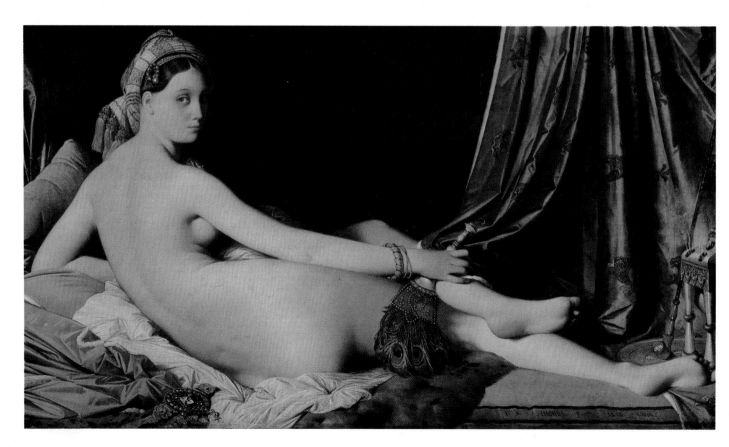

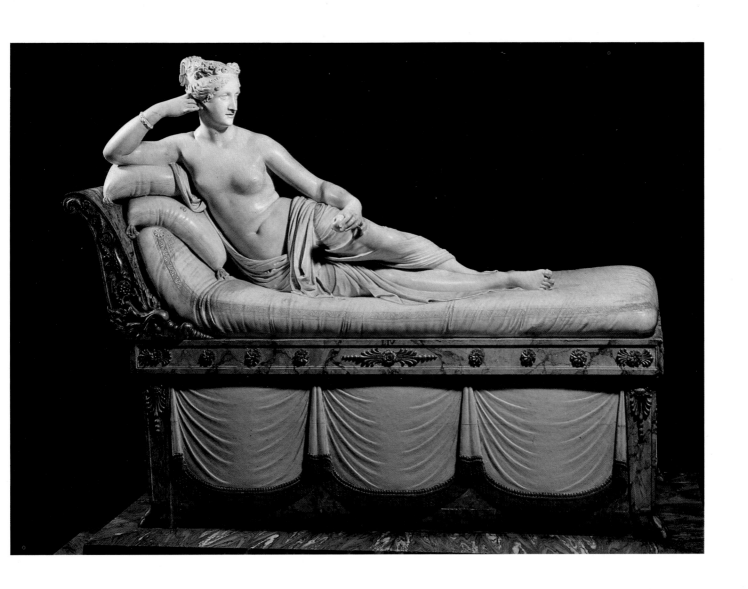

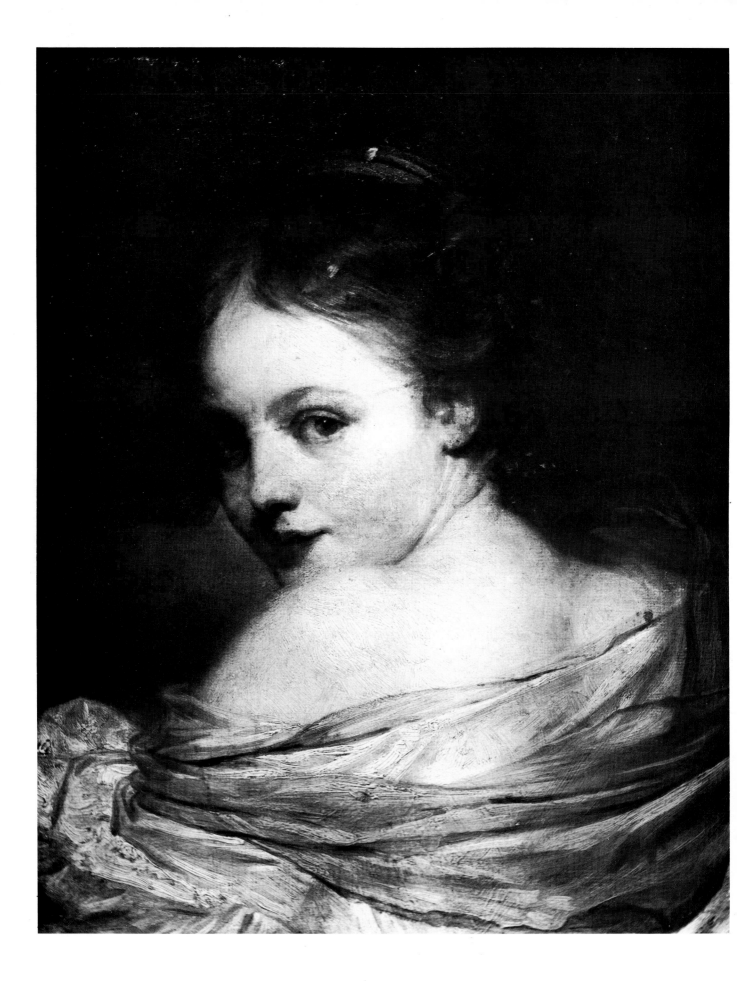

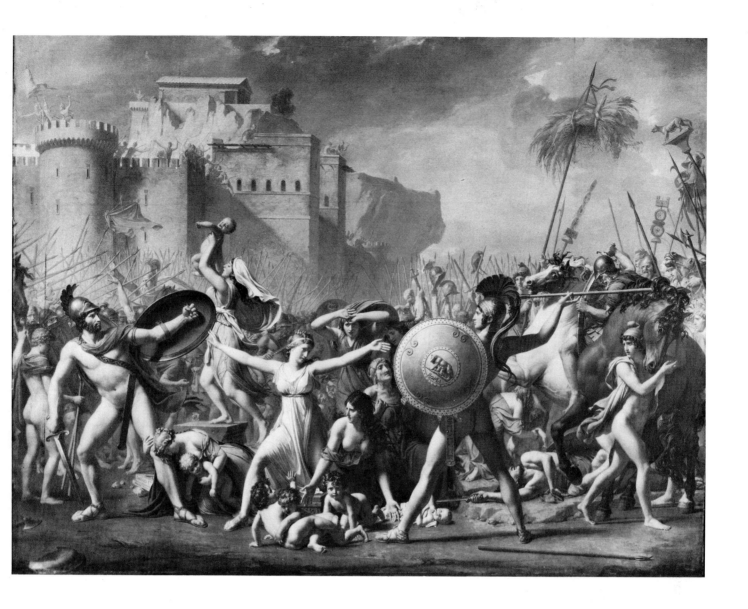

124. PRECEDING PAGES BELOW LEFT Jean-Auguste-Dominique Ingres, *La Grande Odalisque*, 1809
Oil on canvas (Louvre, Paris)

La Grande Odalisque, Ingres' most savagely criticized work, was painted as a pendant to another reclining nude bought by the King of Naples in 1809. The languid pose, the girl's provocative gaze, and the textures of oriental silken trappings make it a painting of incomparable sensuality.

125. OPPOSITE Jean Baptiste Greuze, *Portrait of a Young Girl*
Oil on canvas (Musée de Montpellier)

At the beginning of his long career Greuze was enormously popular, specializing in moralizing narrative subjects such as *The Paralytic Tended by his Children*. But in the 1770s and 1780s the new style of Neo-Classicism gained strength, and to offset his dwindling appeal, Greuze turned to titillatory pictures of half-naked girls.

126. ABOVE Jacques-Louis David, *The Sabine Women*, 1799
Oil on canvas (Louvre, Paris)

David, though brought up in the Rococo world of his distant relative Boucher, quickly turned to Neo-Classicism, and became its best and most celebrated exponent. His involvement in the revolution was political as well as artistic. He voted for the death of Louis XVI, abolished the Academy and, after the fall of Robespierre, was imprisoned. Due to the intercession of his pupils and his wife he was released, and in 1798, partly in recognition of his wife's devotion, and partly as a manifesto of his passion for the antique, he began his painting of the Sabine Women.

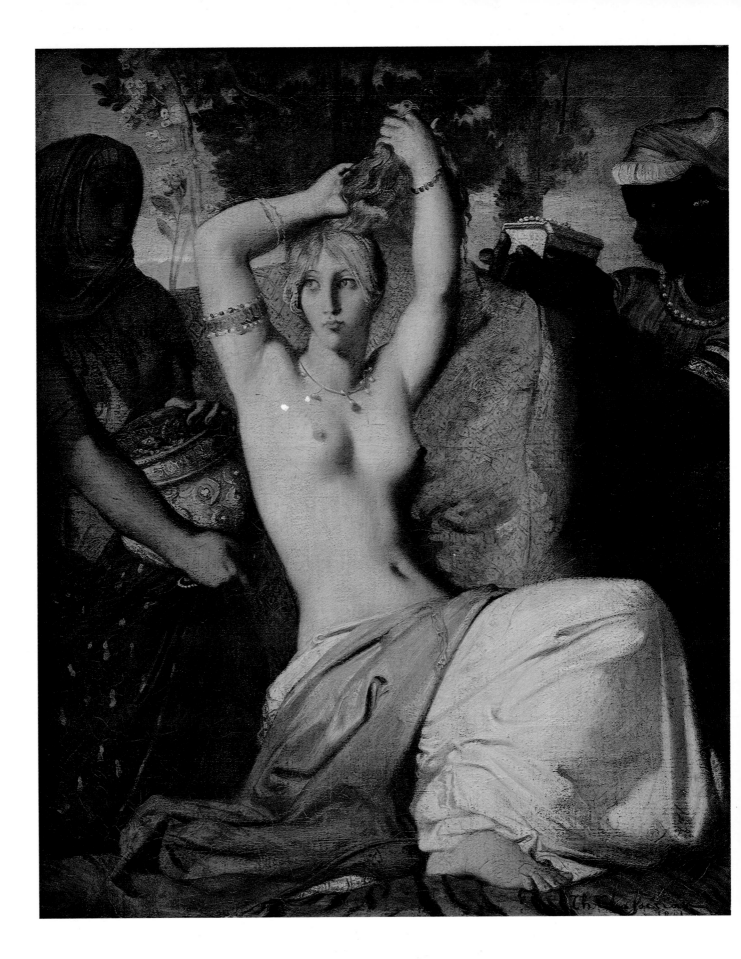

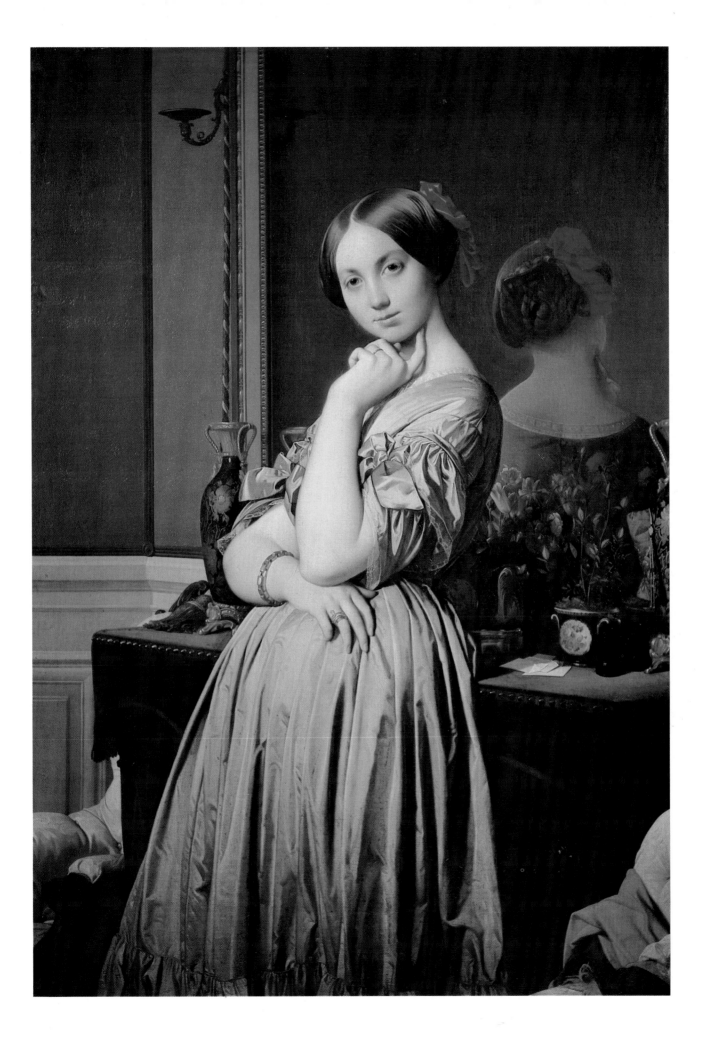

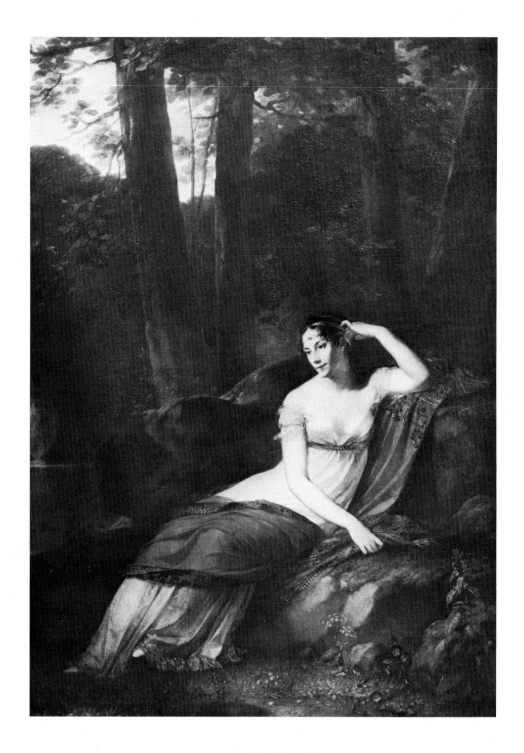

127. PRECEDING PAGES LEFT Théodore Chassériau, *Esther*, 1821
Oil on canvas (Louvre, Paris)

Chassériau, a pupil of Ingres, was also influenced by Delacroix, and, like him, painted many North African scenes, as well as biblical and allegorical subjects. Here, in the story of the beautiful Jewess Esther, he has combined two of his favourite themes. Esther, cousin of Mordecai, married Xerxes, King of the Persian Empire, and successfully pleaded with her husband not to massacre her people throughout his lands, which stretched from Ethiopia to India.

128. PRECEDING PAGES RIGHT Jean-Auguste-Dominique Ingres, *Comtesse d'Haussonville*, 1845
Oil on canvas (Frick Collection, New York)

Louise, Princesse de Broglie, married a diplomat, writer and member of the French Academy, the Comte d'Haussonville, at the age of eighteen. She herself published several books, including a life of Byron. This portrait, for which Ingres made numerous preparatory drawings and which had several false starts, was finally greeted, according to Ingres, with 'a storm of approval'.

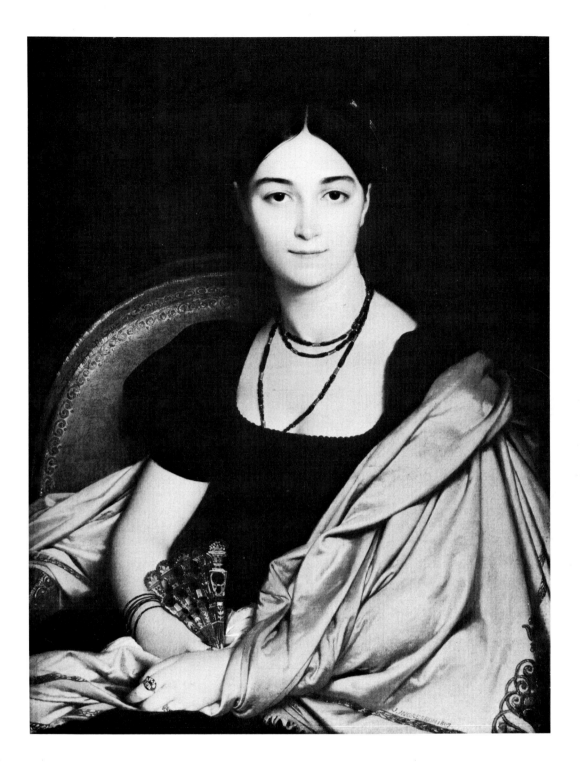

129. OPPOSITE Pierre-Paul Prud'hon, *The Empress Josephine*
Oil on canvas (Louvre, Paris)

Prud'hon was drawing master and Court Painter to the Empress Josephine, and made several portraits of her. His style was individual, more romantic than Neo-Classical, and he was influenced by Raphael, Leonardo and Correggio, as can be seen here. He has portrayed Josephine in a very similar pose to that of her sister-in-law, Paolina Borghese, in Canova's marble sculpture of 1808.

130. ABOVE Jean-Auguste-Dominique Ingres, *Madame Devauçay*, 1807
Oil on canvas (Musée Condé, Chantilly)

This portrait, which Ingres did shortly after his arrival in Rome, is in many ways similar to one of Madame Rivière that he painted in France in 1805. The same emphasis is given to the face by placing it in front of a completely plain, dark background, while the main area of decoration is an embroidered cashmere shawl.

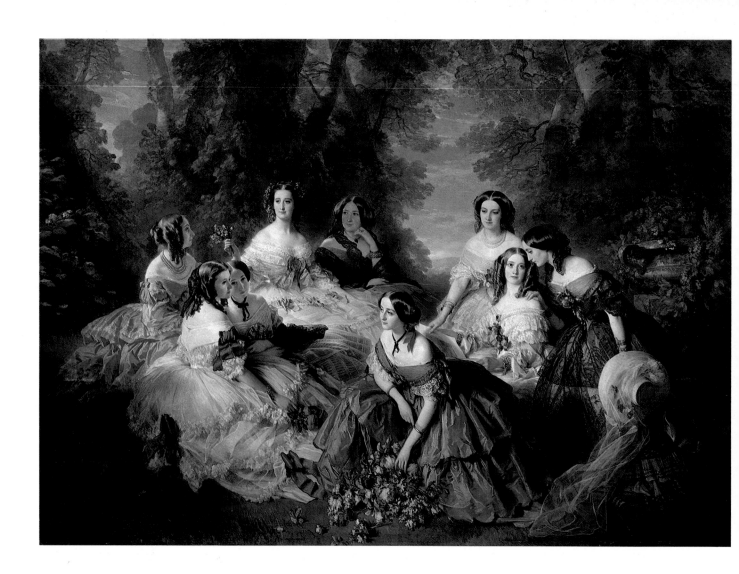

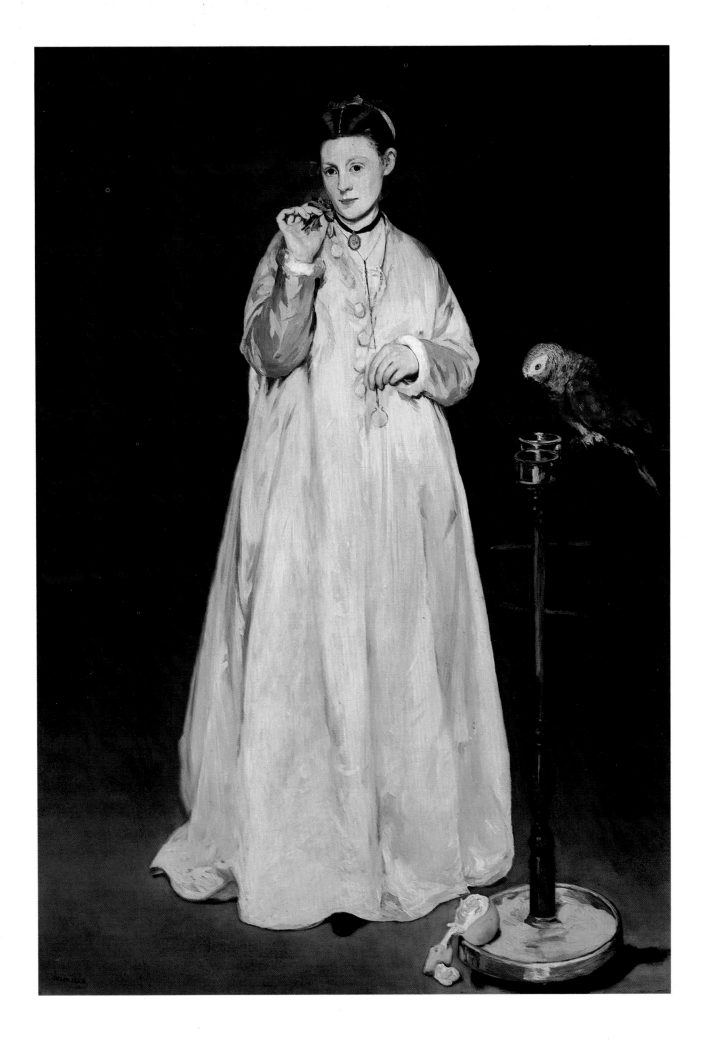

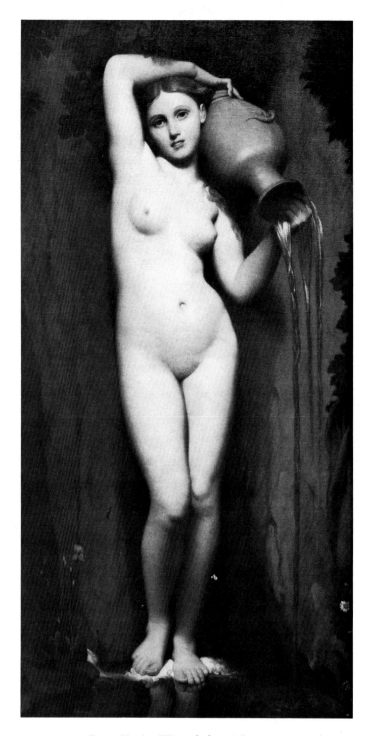

131. PRECEDING PAGES LEFT Franz Xavier Winterhalter, *The Empress Eugénie Accompanied by her Ladies-in-Waiting*, 1855
Oil on canvas (Musée de Compiègne)

When the Spanish Eugénie de Montijo married Napoleon III, she brought with her a style of court life unknown in France for over a hundred years. She and her retinue of ladies-in-waiting, drawn from the aristocracies of Spain and France, spent much of their time at the Palace of Fontainebleau, where often the house parties were so large that guests had to be lodged at a local hotel.

132. PRECEDING PAGES RIGHT Edouard Manet, *Woman with a Parrot*, 1866
Oil on canvas (Metropolitan Museum of Art, New York: Gift of Erwin Davis, 1889)

Woman with a Parrot has been interpreted as an allegory of the five senses, in which the parrot symbolizes the sense of hearing, while the peeled orange, the violets, the fingered ribbon and the monocle portray respectively the senses of taste, smell, touch and sight. The woman is Manet's favourite model, Victorine Meurent.

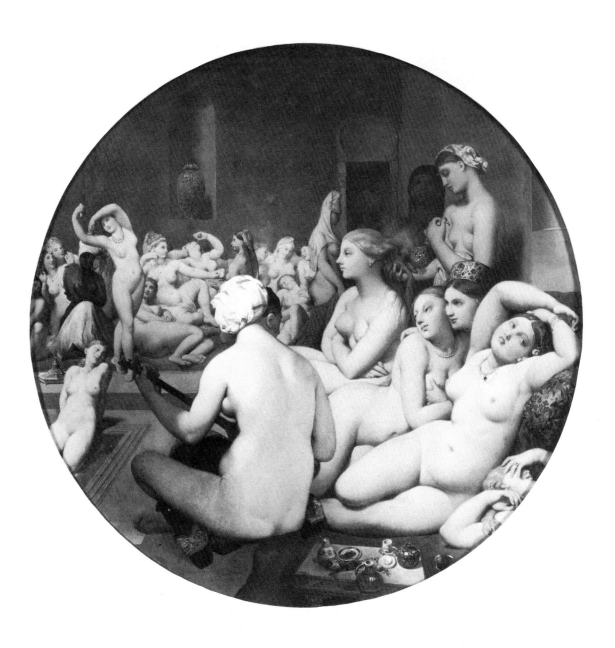

133. OPPOSITE Jean-Auguste-Dominique Ingres, *La Source*, 1856
Oil on canvas (Louvre, Paris)

Ingres began studies for a painting based on Botticelli's *Venus* as early as 1817. He completed one version of the idea, the *Venus Anadyomene*, in 1848, and eight years later he painted *La Source*, adapting the figure of Venus into a girl carrying a pitcher. *La Source* was immediately popular and has been called the most beautiful figure in French painting.

134. ABOVE Jean-Auguste-Dominique Ingres, *Le Bain Turc*, 1862
Oil on canvas (Louvre, Paris)

Ideas connected with this work engaged Ingres during the year 1827–8, when he seems to have achieved a satisfactory solution: but the actual picture is dated 1862. Most of the figures had occupied his imagination during these years, in particular the back view of a woman playing a mandolin, which is a version of his most beautiful work the *Baigneuse de Valpinçon*. *Le Bain Turc* is an extreme example of the economy with which Ingres used his small but priceless store of ideas.

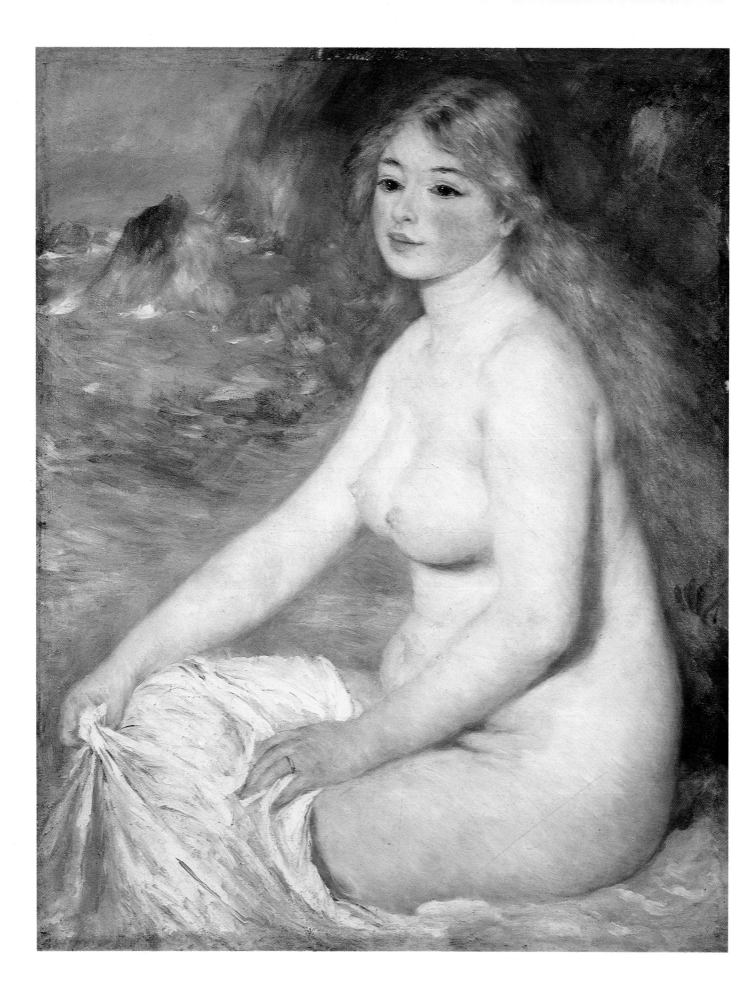

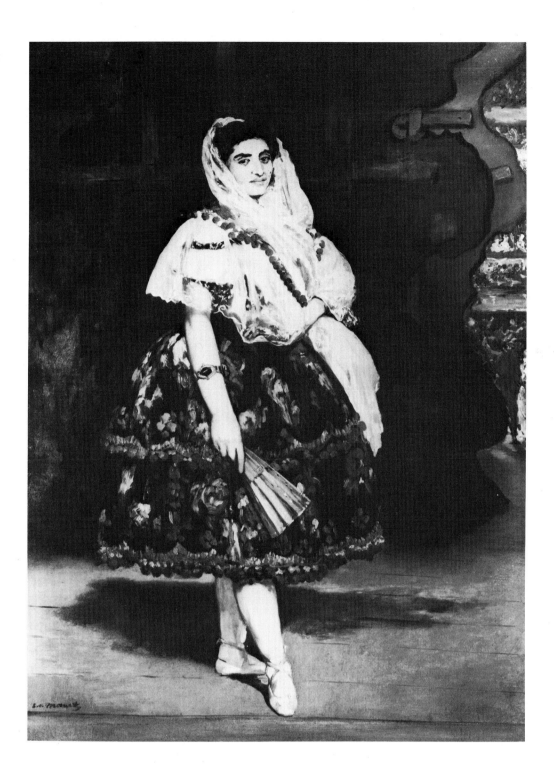

135. OPPOSITE Pierre-Auguste Renoir, *Blonde Bather*, 1881
Oil on canvas (Sterling and Francine Clark Institute, Williamstown, Massachusetts)

The artist's wife was the model for the dazzling *Blonde Bather*, painted during a trip to Italy in 1881.
It is said that Renoir began work on this picture in a boat in the Bay of Naples, in the full
Mediterranean sunlight.

136. ABOVE Edouard Manet, *Lola de Valence*, 1862
Oil on canvas (Louvre, Paris)

Manet's admiration for the Spanish school in painting receives general expression in this tribute to a
popular contemporary dancer. A member of the Camprubi ballet company, Lola de Valence was
the toast of the 1862 season at the Paris Hippodrome. She is posed, in full costume, in the wings of
the stage.

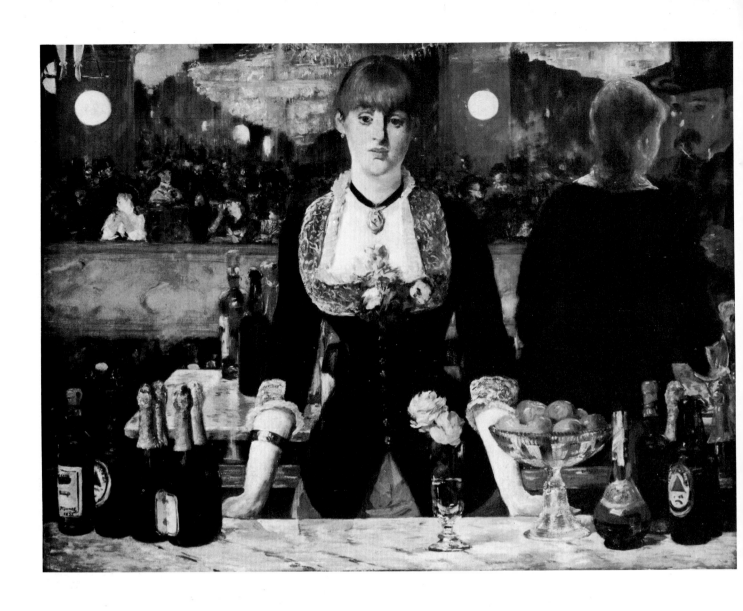

137. Edouard Manet, *The Bar at the Folies-Bergères*, 1881–2
Oil on canvas (Courtauld Institute Galleries, London)

Besides making numerous studies on the spot for *The Bar at the Folies-Bergères*, Manet arranged for a
model of the bar itself to be constructed in his studio. The painting, now one of his most admired,
was first exhibited at the 1882 Salon, and immediately attracted criticism as a wilful deviation from
accepted artistic standards. One critic singled it out as an example of 'the intrusion of banal and
vulgar scenes of contemporary life into the field of serious painting'.

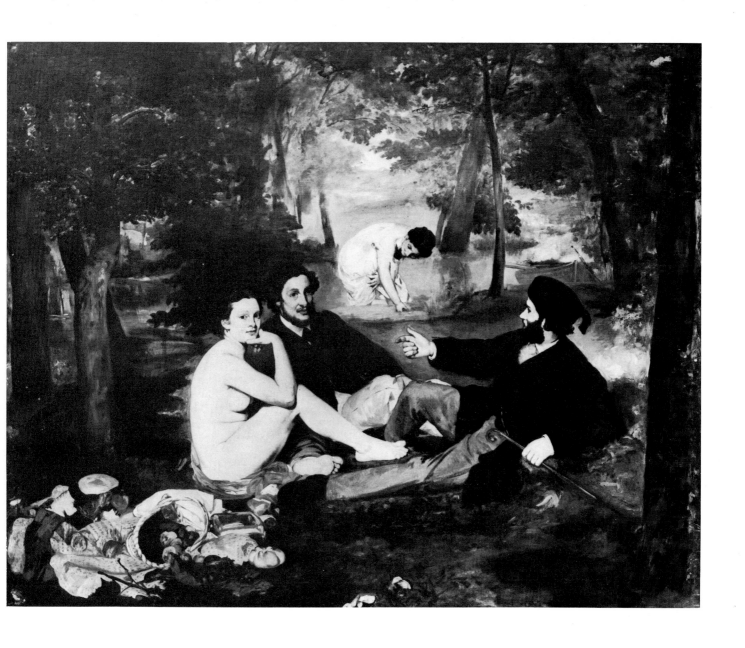

138. Edouard Manet, *Le Déjeuner sur l'Herbe*, 1862–3
Oil on canvas (Jeu de Paume, Paris)

Once again, Manet offended prevailing artistic tastes by taking an accepted formula, in this case
based on a Marcantonio engraving after Raphael and Giorgione's *Concert Champêtre*, and
interpreting it with uncompromising modernism. Victorine Meurent is shown here enjoying a
highly unconventional picnic with Manet's brother, Eugène, and future brother-in-law, Ferdinand.
When visiting the Salon for the 1863 exhibition in which *Le Déjeuner sur l'Herbe* was first shown,
Napoleon III is reputed to have turned away with a gesture indicating that he considered the
painting an affront to public morality.

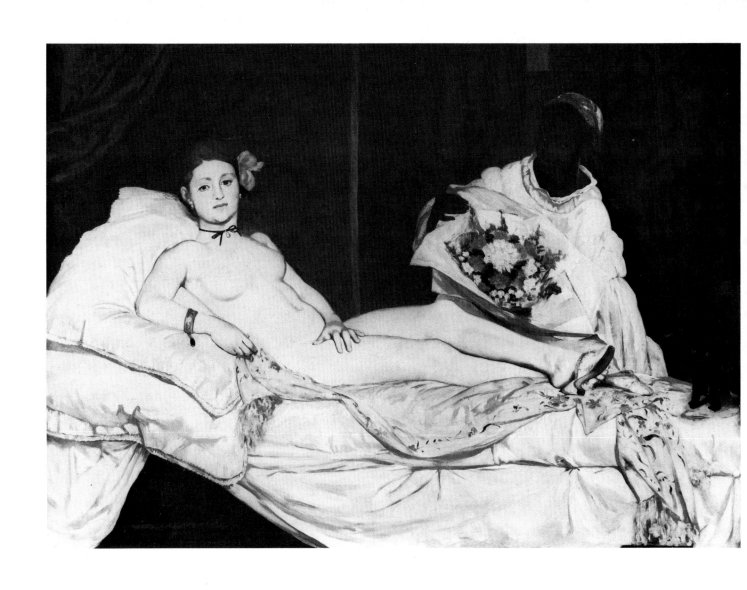

139. Edouard Manet, *Olympia*, 1863
Oil on canvas (Jeu de Paume, Paris)

The pictorial motif of the reclining nude and attendant servant is recurrent in art, but Manet's
decision to interpret the subject in modern terms provoked a scandalized outcry. His
demi-mondaine, with her frank gaze and exotic companions, was the sensation of the 1865 Salon. Not
all were blind to its merits at the time, however: Cézanne admired the painting greatly and
Gauguin made a copy of it.

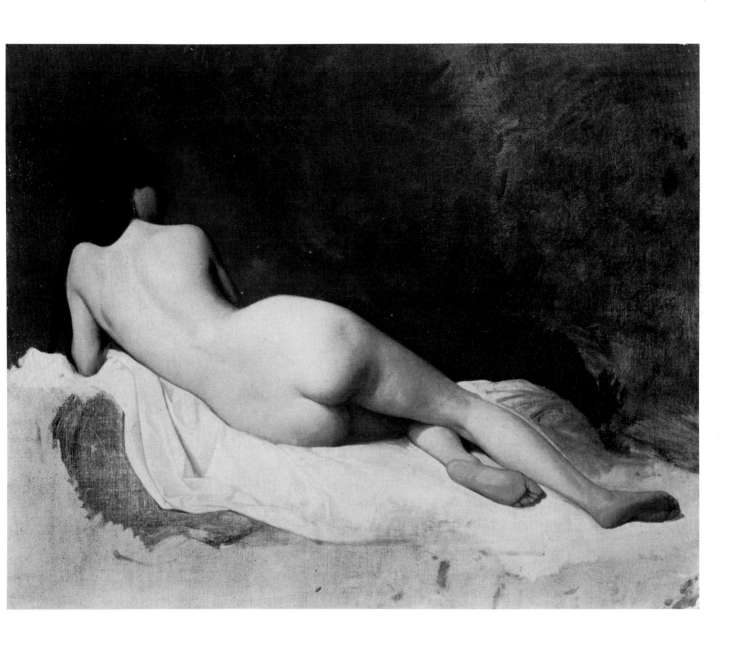

140. Thomas Couture, *Odalisque*
Oil on canvas (Cleveland Museum of Art, Ohio)

A synthesis of Neo-Classicism and Romanticism, Couture's erotic linear nude is another example of
the reclining odalisque, a popular theme in the nineteenth-century. An artist and a teacher,
Couture's most celebrated pupil was Manet.

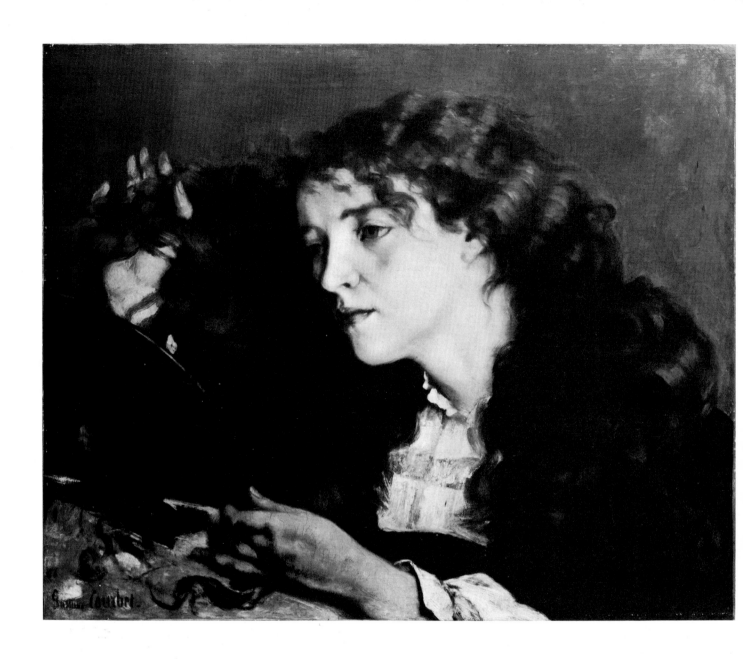

141. ABOVE Gustave Courbet, *Jo, la belle Irlandaise*, 1866
Oil on canvas (Nationalmuseum, Stockholm)

Long hair became something of a fetish in nineteenth-century art, and the luxuriant tresses of many of the century's *femmes fatales* seem to be as much a weapon as an adornment. Here, Courbet's Irish beauty examines her abundant auburn curls.

142. OPPOSITE George Frederic Watts, *Choosing*, 1864
Oil on canvas (National Portrait Gallery, London)

Watts painted his girl-bride, the actress Ellen Terry, just before her seventeenth birthday in her wedding dress, which was designed by Holman Hunt. She is smelling a scentless camellia, a pose which has caused some controversy.

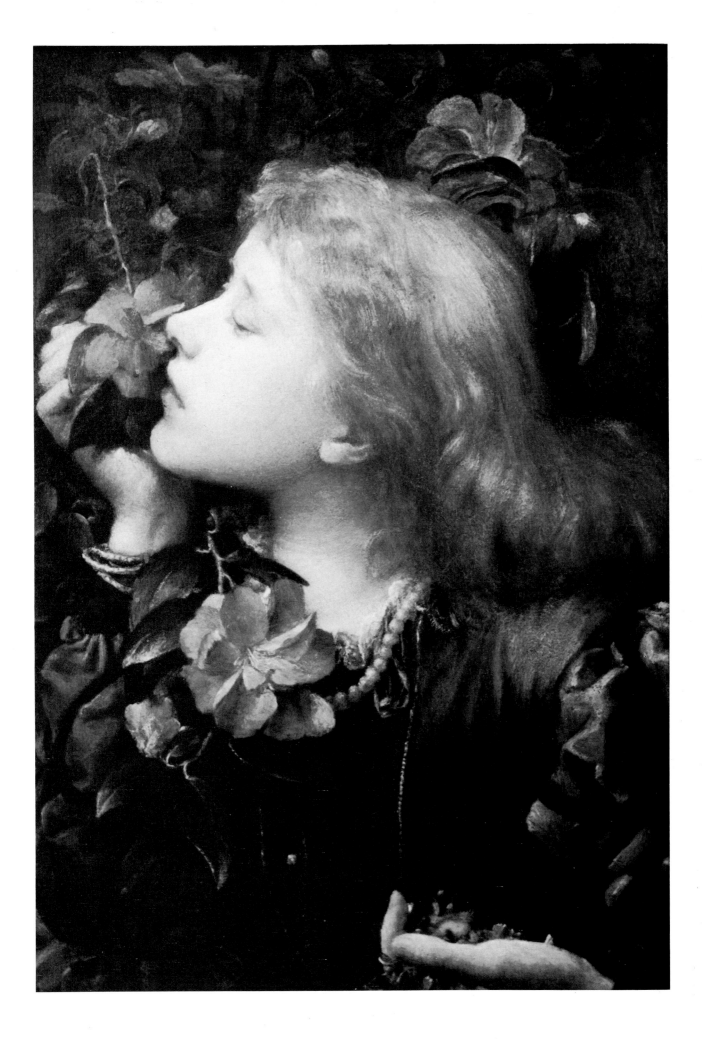

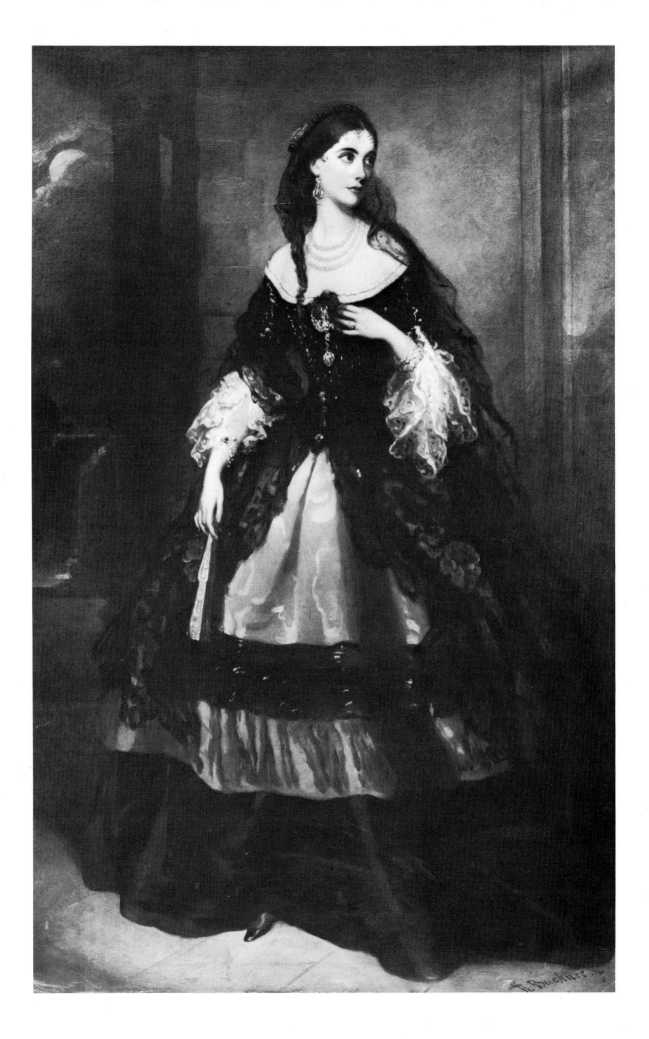

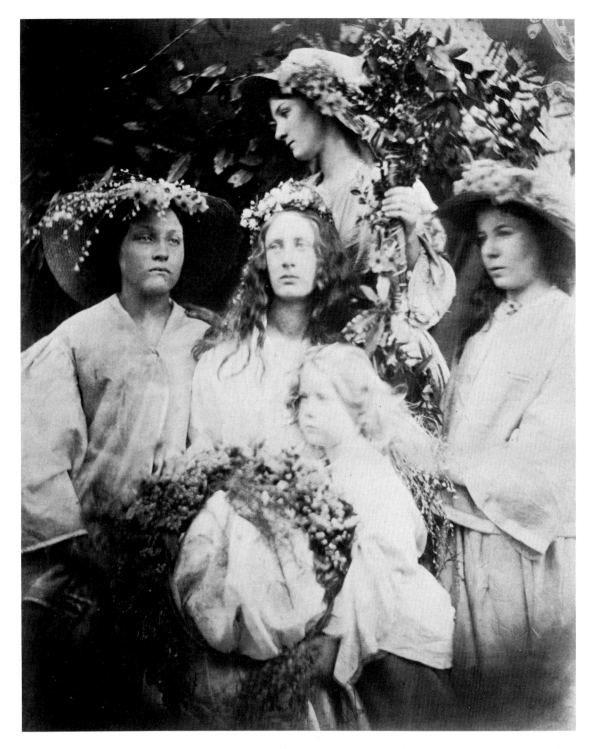

143. OPPOSITE Richard Buckner, *Countess of Cardigan*
Oil on canvas (Private Collection)

A celebrated nineteenth-century beauty, Miss Horsey de Horsey, scandalized society by flaunting her friendship with the married Lord Cardigan of Balaclava fame. Eventually she became his second wife and, even when she married again after his death, she continued to display both his uniform and the stuffed head of his charger in her front hall.

144. ABOVE Julia Margaret Cameron, *Rosebud Garden of Girls*, 1868
Photograph (Royal Photographic Society, London)

Mrs Cameron, who took up photography in middle age, was completely self-taught. She is famous for portraits of her illustrious friends – Darwin, Herschel, Tennyson, Carlyle, Browning and Longfellow – and for seemingly natural but in fact painstakingly posed photographs of romanticized girls, though she seems occasionally to have run out of beauties.

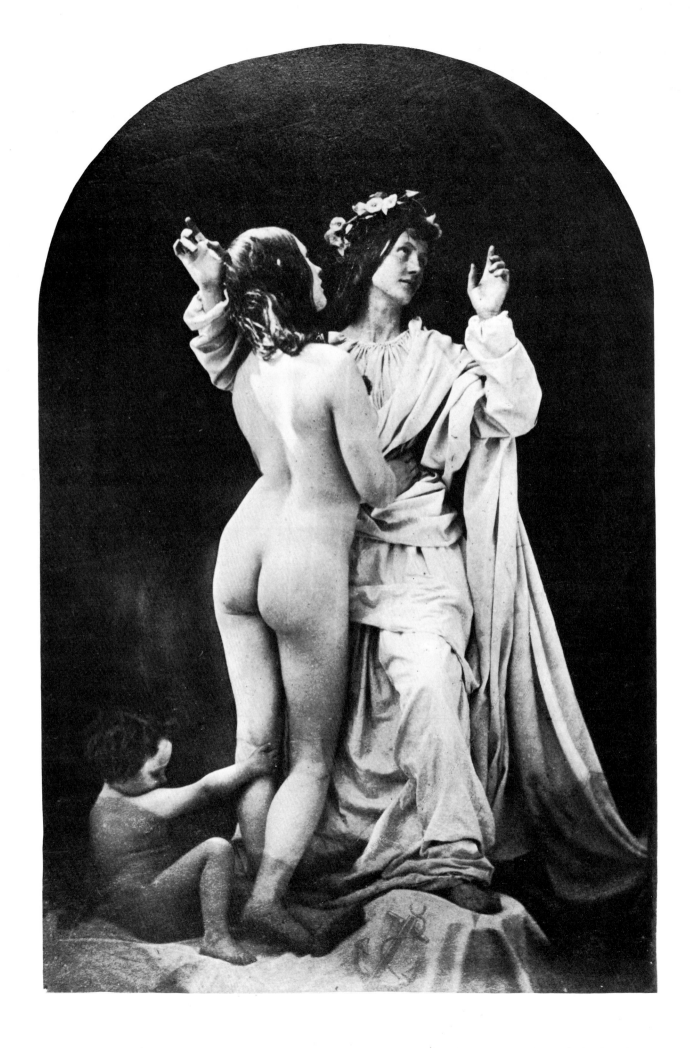

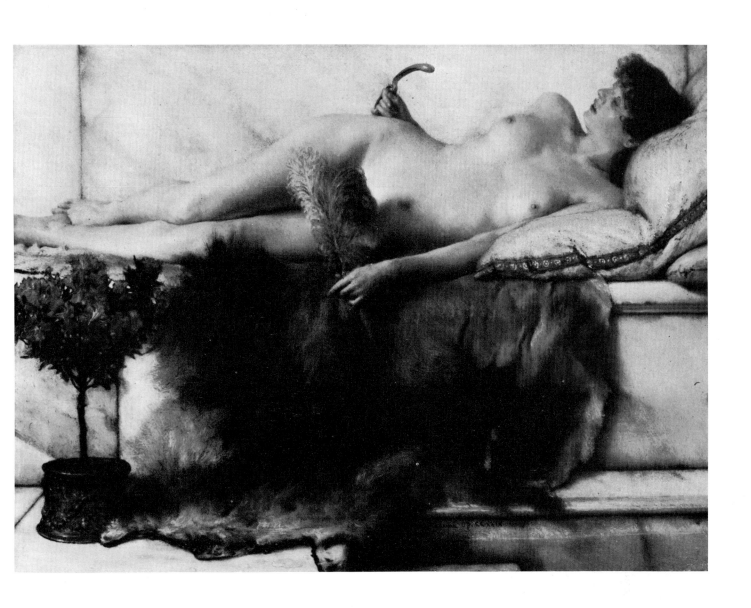

145. OPPOSITE Oscar Gustave Rejlander, *Two Women and a Child, c.* 1855
Photograph (Mansell Collection, London)

Rejlander popularized in London his own brand of staged 'art photography', frequently taking a
theme from the Bible or duplicating a successful academic painting.

146. ABOVE Sir Lawrence Alma-Tadema, *In the Tepidarium*, 1881
Oil on canvas (Lady Lever Art Gallery, Port Sunlight)

A leading Royal Academican, Alma-Tadema produced glowing reconstructions of ancient Greek
and Roman life that were extremely popular in the nineteenth century. The unabashed sensuality of
this painting escaped attack from Victorian critics because the reclining nude figure has certain
classical trappings. Langorously posed in the ante-chamber of a Roman bath, Alma-Tadema's
model holds a strigil or body scraper in one hand and, more fancifully, an ostrich feather fan
in the other.

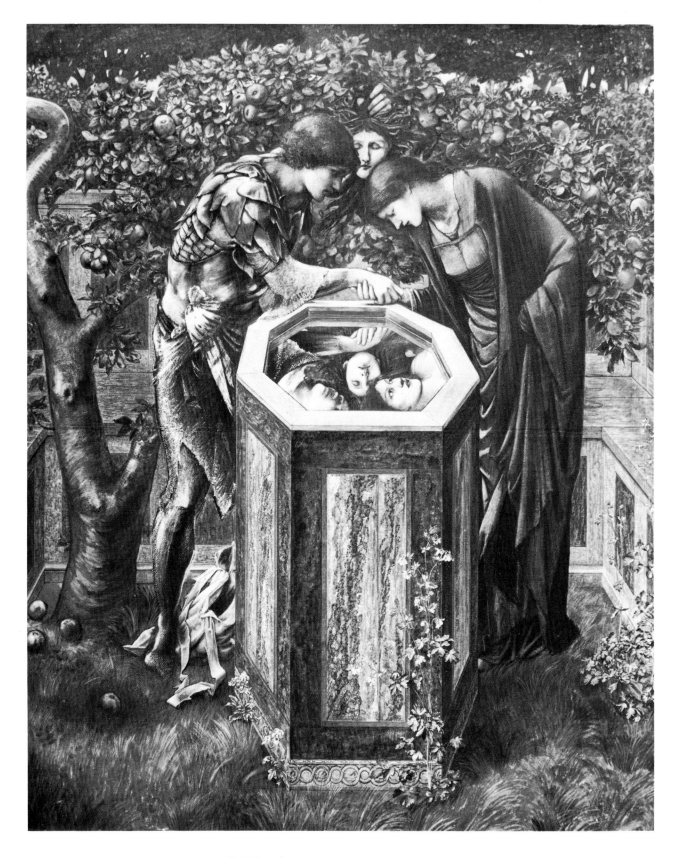

147. Sir Edward Burne-Jones, *Perseus and his Bride, c.* 1885
Gouache (Southampton Art Gallery)

Burne-Jones' famous Perseus series was commissioned by Arthur Balfour in 1875 to decorate his music-room. Unfortunately the cycle of paintings was never completed, but full-scale gouache cartoons for each were prepared. Here, Perseus shows his wife Andromeda the head of the Medusa reflected in a well. The Vorticist artist Wyndham Lewis was a keen admirer of the series, in which he saw elements of pioneer surrealism.

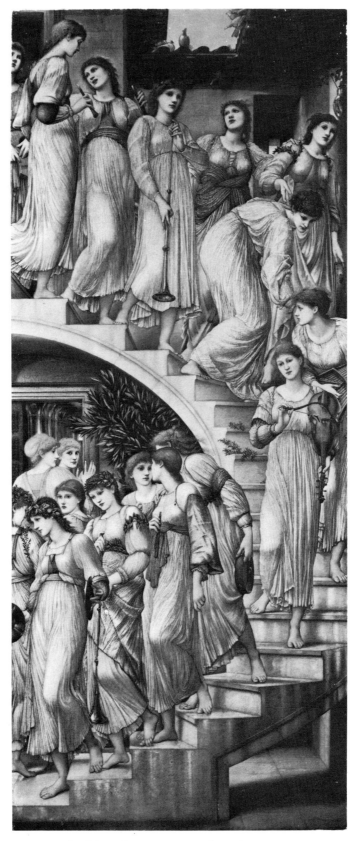

148. Sir Edward Burne-Jones, *The Golden Stairs*, 1880
Oil on canvas (Tate Gallery, London)

Contemporaries were disconcerted by the absence of any explicit subject in this painting, and, according to Lady Burne-Jones, the artist received 'many letters from different parts of the world asking for an explanation'. Apparently involved in some arcane ceremonial, Burne-Jones' descending nymphs have a mysterious remoteness which is intensified by the painting's formal classicism.

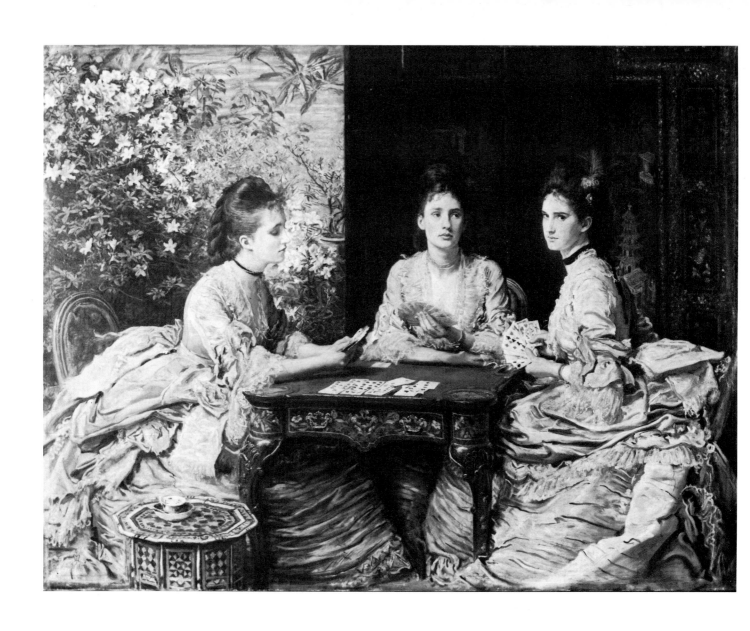

149. Sir John Everett Millais, *Hearts are Trumps*, 1872
Oil on canvas (Tate Gallery, London)

Walter Armstrong's three daughters, Elizabeth, Diana and Mary, in dresses designed by Millais,
play dummy whist in this group portrait. First exhibited at the Royal Academy, the painting was
much admired by the critics. One wrote: 'the painting is as brilliant, lucid and forcible as
Velazquez, and as broad as Reynolds. It contains what, on the whole, are the best portraits Mr
Millais has produced . . . it will be among the most powerful attractions of this year's Exhibition.'

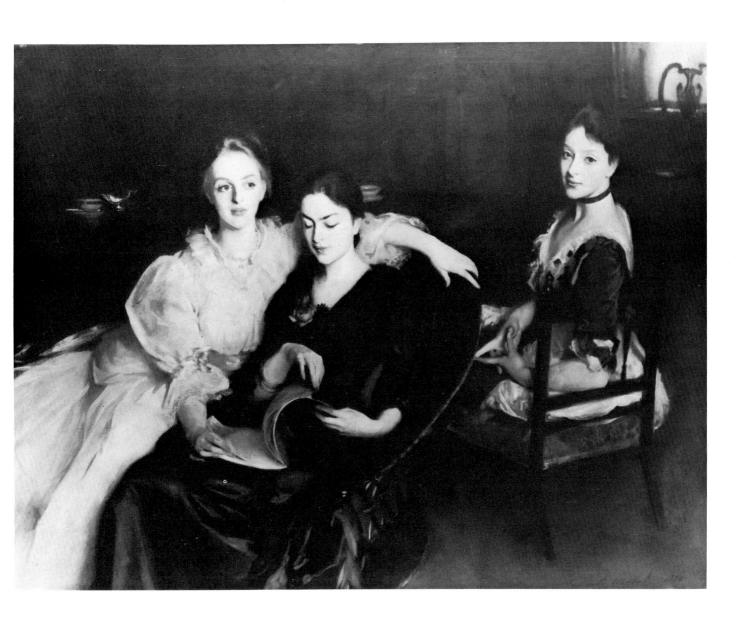

150. John Singer Sargent, *The Misses Vickers*, 1884
Oil on canvas (Sheffield City Art Galleries)

Sargent's many portraits have left a vivid record of the values of an opulent and self-confident age
in which the *nouveaux riches* were elevated to the ranks of high society. This group portrait was
commissioned by Colonel Thomas Vickers, head of the Sheffield engineering firm. His daughters,
'three ugly young women' as Sargent described them in a letter to a friend, are imbued here with
considerable charm.

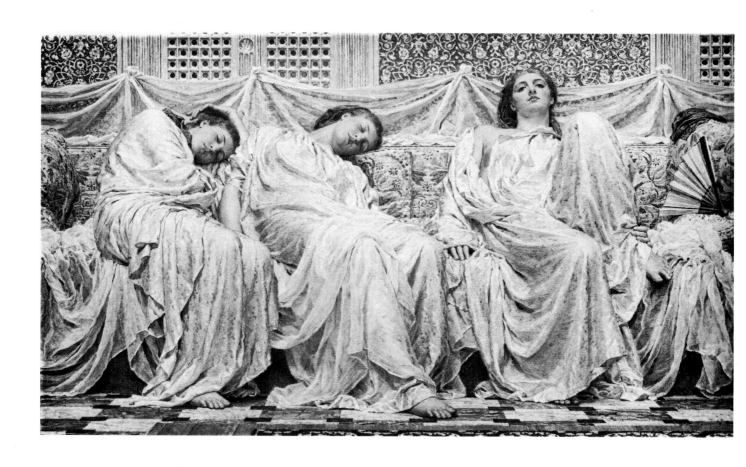

151. ABOVE Albert Moore, *Dreamers*, 1882
Oil on canvas (Birmingham City Museums and Art Gallery)

The aesthetic philosophy of analogies between painting and music was reflected in Albert Moore's fascination with colour harmonies. His paintings celebrated an imaginary Antique lifestyle, often 'modernized' with conspicuously anachronistic references, such as the Japonnaiseries here. Themes of sleeping and dreaming recurred in Moore's work as the artist consciously tried to eliminate all expressive elements from his subject matter.

152. OPPOSITE Lord Leighton, *Flaming June*, c. 1895
Oil on canvas (Museo de Arte de Ponce, Puerto Rico)

Leighton is best remembered for pictures capturing the idealized delights of a vanished Olympian world. His careful preparations for finished paintings involved study sketches of the models, both nude and draped, and often the modelling of small statuettes of individual figures in order to achieve greater authenticity. *Flaming June* was painted while the artist was suffering from his final illness, the year before his death in 1896.

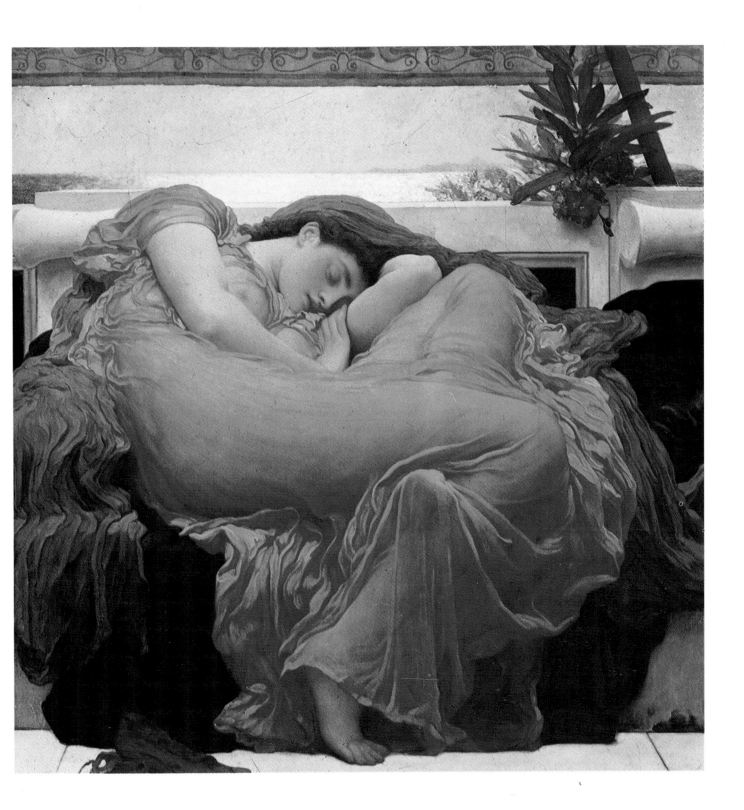

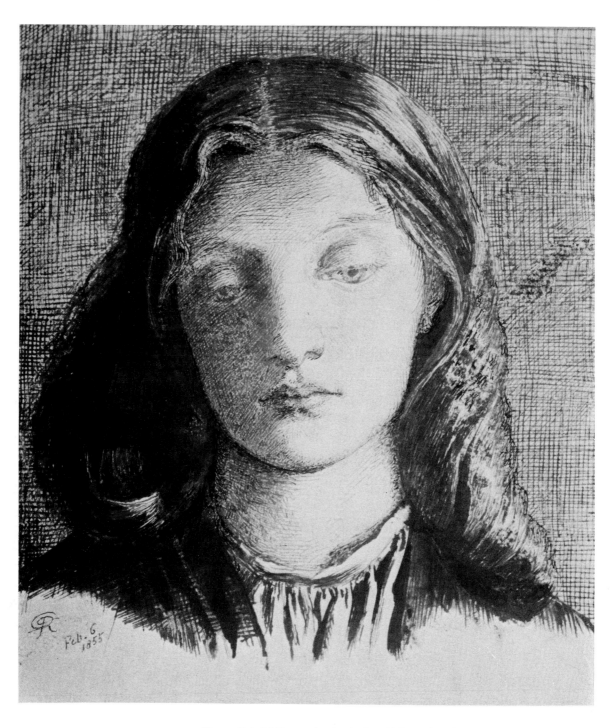

153. ABOVE Dante Gabriel Rossetti, *Elizabeth Siddal*, 6 February, 1855
Pen and brown and black ink (Ashmolean Museum, Oxford: F.F. Madan Bequest)

From 1851 'Lizzie' Siddal, or 'Guggums' as she was affectionately nicknamed by the other
Pre-Raphaelites, began to sit exclusively for Rossetti, and was his chief inspiration for the next
eleven years, until her death in 1862. Visiting Rossetti on 6 October 1854, Madox Brown recorded:
'saw Miss Siddal, looking thinner and more deathlike and more beautiful and more ragged than
ever . . . Gabriel . . . drawing wonderful and lovely Guggums one after another, each one stamped
with immortality.'

154. OPPOSITE *Jane Morris*, 1865
Photograph (Victoria and Albert Museum, London)

This photograph of Jane Morris was posed by Rossetti in the garden of his house in Chelsea in July
1865, and was used as a preliminary study for his painting *The Reverie*. Jane Morris typified
Rossetti's feminine ideal, with her long neck, strikingly voluptuous features and thick waving hair,
and became the artist's favourite model following the death of Elizabeth Siddal.

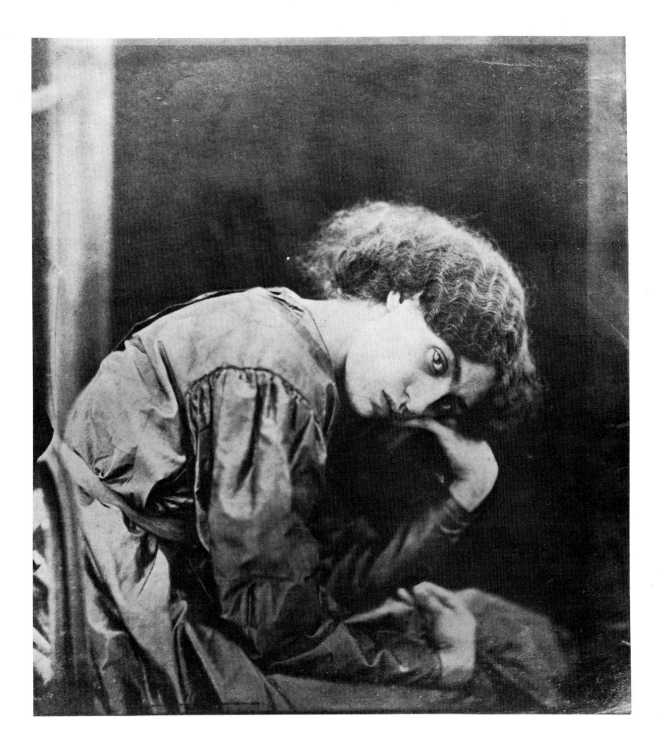

155. OVERLEAF LEFT Dante Gabriel Rossetti, *The Angel Gabriel Appearing to the Virgin Mary*, 1850
Oil on canvas (Tate Gallery, London)

One of Rossetti's earliest Pre-Raphaelite paintings, this unconventional interpretation of the
Annunciation aroused such strong criticism at its first showing, at the Portland Gallery in London,
that the artist subsequently refused an invitation to exhibit the picture in Liverpool, and thereafter
showed his work in London as little as possible.

156. OVERLEAF RIGHT Dante Gabriel Rossetti, *Beata Beatrix*, c. 1862/3–70
Oil on canvas (Tate Gallery, London)

Rossetti began *Beata Beatrix* shortly after the suicide of his wife, Lizzie Siddal. It is a tribute to her,
not only as an outstandingly beautiful portrait but also in its subject matter: she is cast in the role of
one of history's most famous women, Dante's Beatrice. In a letter to Lady Mount Temple (who
bought the picture) Rossetti wrote 'you are well acquainted with Dante's *Vita Nuova* which
illustrates symbolically the death of Beatrice'.

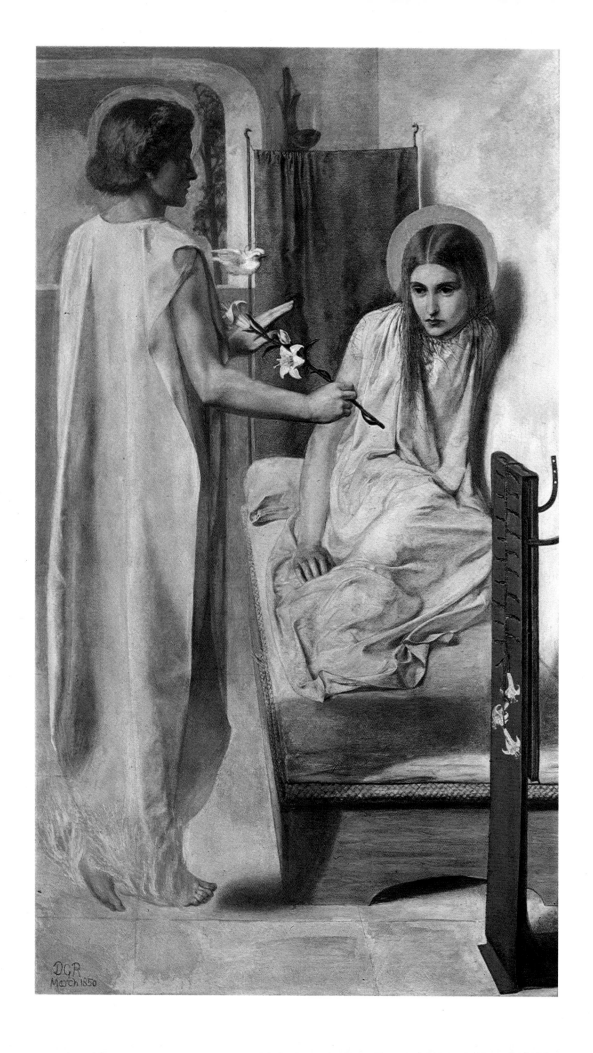

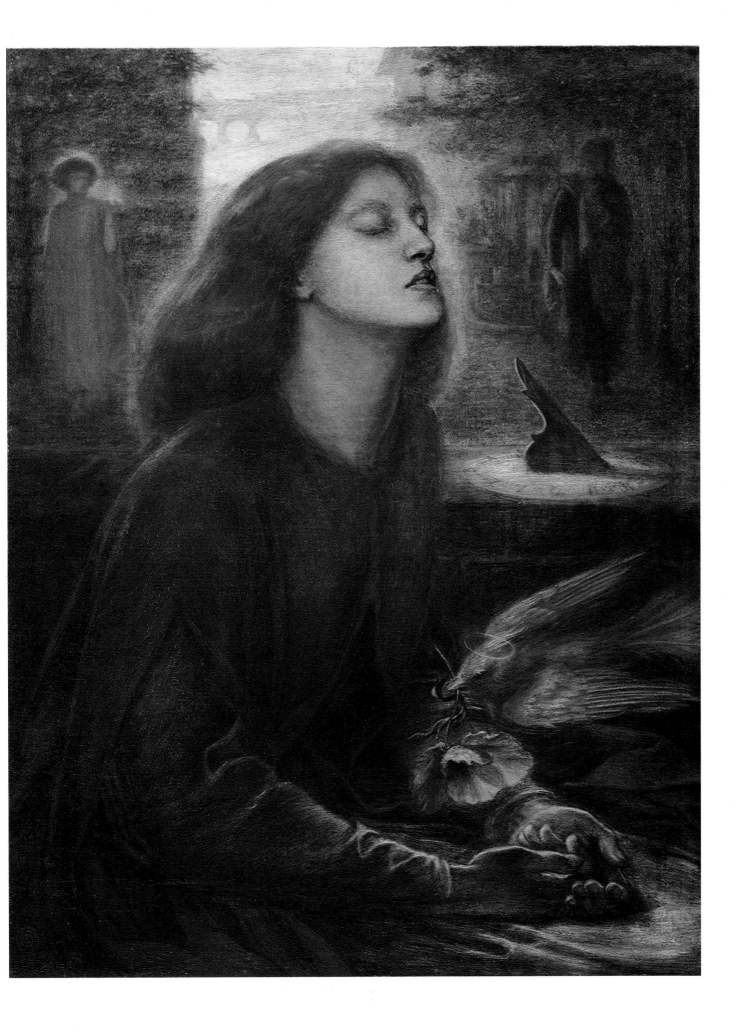

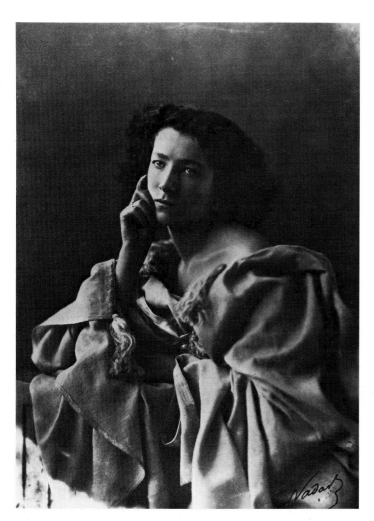 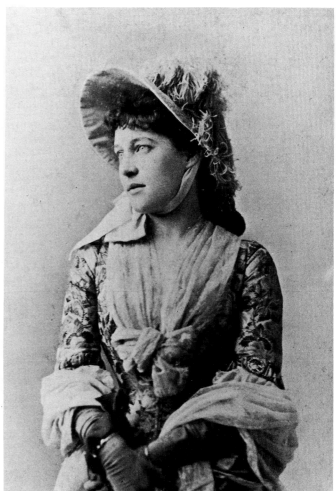

157. ABOVE LEFT Gaspard Felix Tournachon (Nadar), *Sarah Bernhardt*, 1859
Photograph (Bibliothèque Nationale, Paris)

This photograph of the young and beautiful Sarah Bernhardt was taken in 1859, at the start of her dazzling career. In the same year a critic, reviewing an exhibition of photographs by Nadar, wrote in the Gazette des Beaux-Arts: 'All the artistic, dramatic, political galaxy – in a word the intelligentsia – of Paris has passed through his studio.'

158. ABOVE RIGHT *Lily Langtry*
Photograph (Mansell Collection, London)

Lily Langtry, the darling of the London stage and the mistress of the Prince of Wales, photographed in New York. Her face has a glowing sweetness that gave rise to her nickname of the Jersey Lily.

159. OPPOSITE *Lily Langtry with Sarah Bernhardt*
Photograph (Mansell Collection, London)

The two most famous women of their day, photographed together, make an intriguing contrast of worlds, looks and styles.

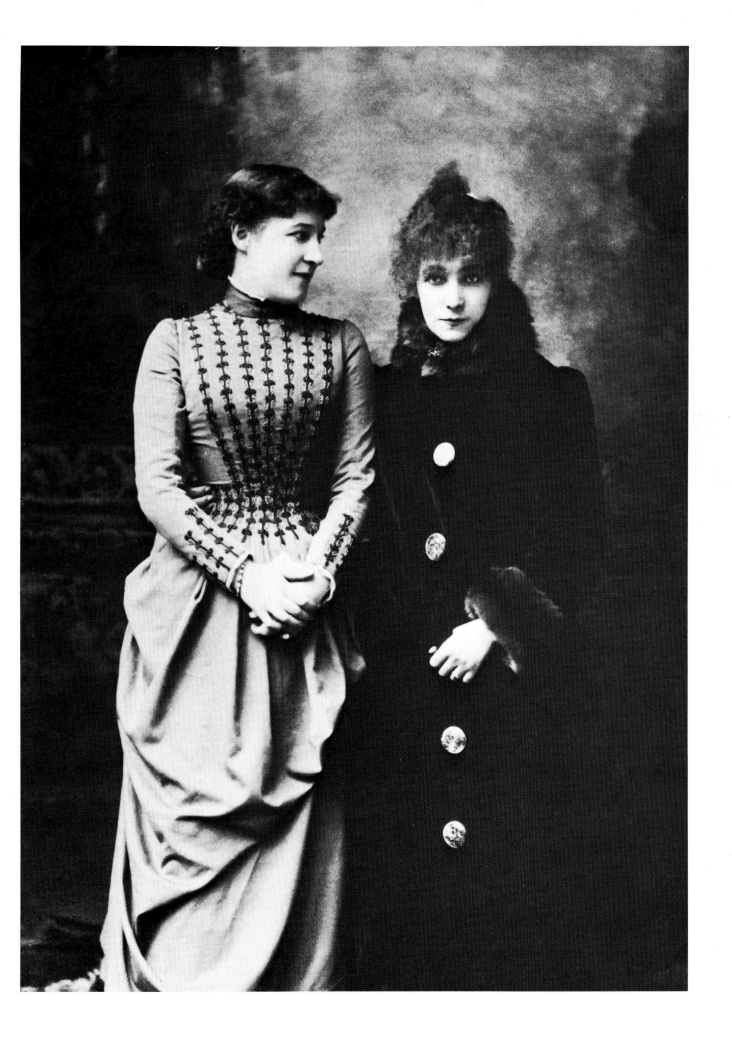

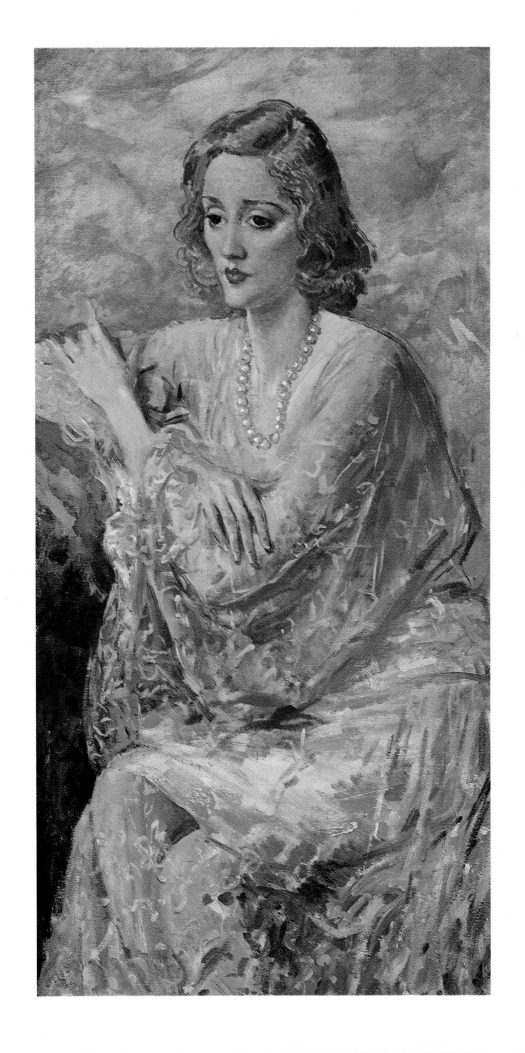

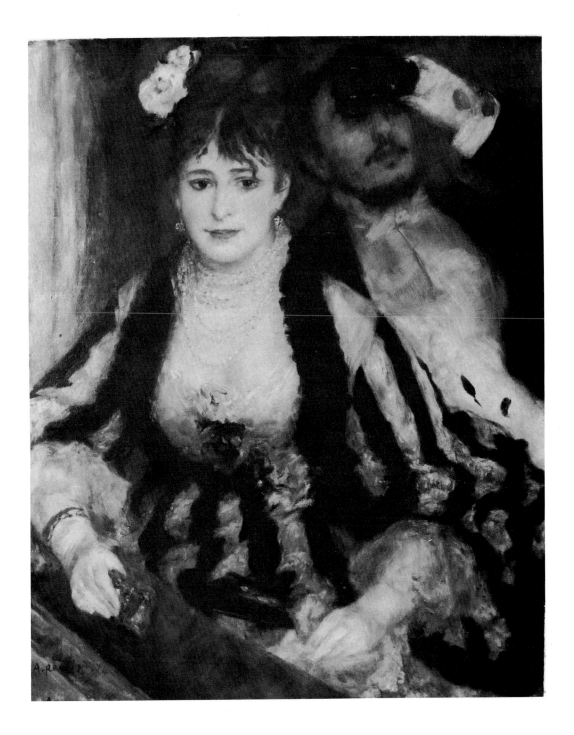

160. OPPOSITE Augustus John, *Tallulah Bankhead*, 1930
Oil on canvas (National Portrait Gallery, Smithsonian Institution, Washington DC: Gift of the
Honourable and Mrs John Hay Whitney)

The American actress Tallulah Bankhead reached the climax of her London career in *He's Mine*,
which opened in October 1929. Augustus John asked her to sit for him in 1930. She accepted on
condition that he sold the portrait to her for £1,000 after it had been exhibited at the Royal
Academy. It was her most prized possession, and hung in the bedroom of every house she lived in.

161. ABOVE Pierre-Auguste Renoir, *La Loge*, 1874
Oil on canvas (Courtauld Institute Galleries, London)

La Loge, exhibited at the historic first Impressionist show in 1874, is one of the series of richly-
coloured, exuberant paintings of the social scene for which Renoir is best known today. A new
model, Nini, posed for the elegant young girl, while Renoir's younger brother Edmond took the
part of her theatre companion. Desperate for money to pay the rent. Renoir persuaded the dealer
Père Martin to buy the painting for 425 francs.

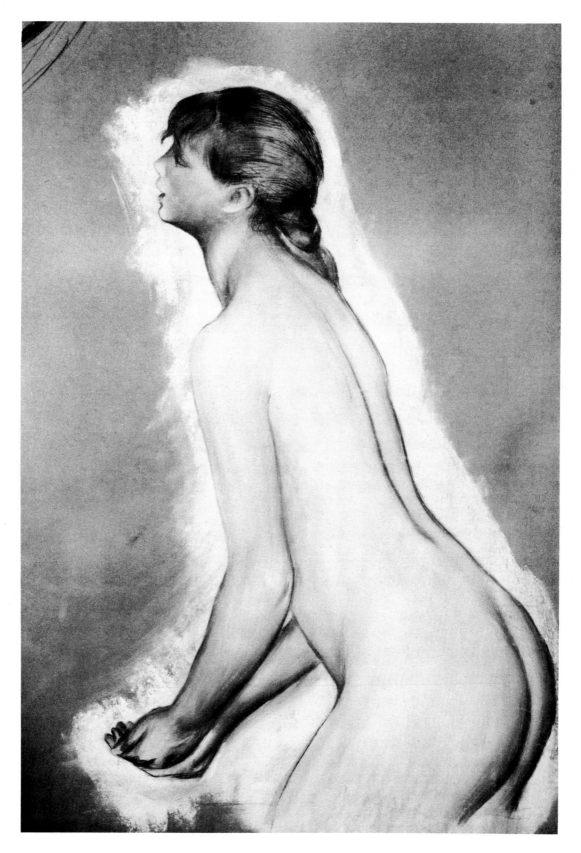

162. Pierre-Auguste Renoir, Study for *The Bathers*, *c.* 1887
Charcoal (Art Institute of Chicago)

Renoir made several delightful studies for *The Bathers*, of which this is one. The finished painting
lacked the more decorative romanticism of his earlier work and received a mixed reaction when it
was first exhibited at the George Petit Gallery in Paris in 1887. Suzanne Valadon, model to Renoir,
Degas and Toulouse-Lautrec, who subsequently established herself as an artist in her own right,
posed for the final version.

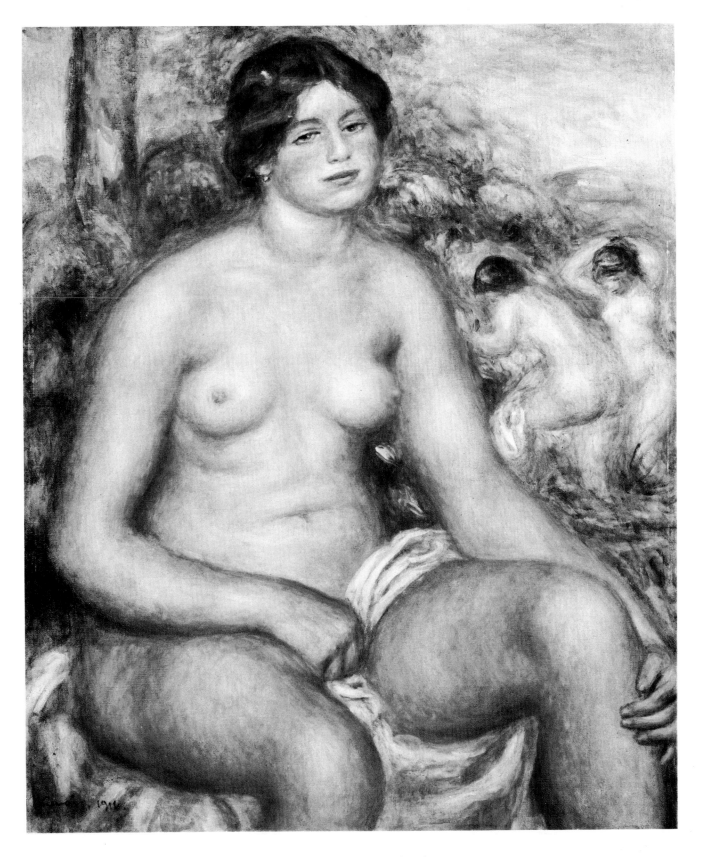

163. Pierre-Auguste Renoir, *Seated Nude*, 1916
Oil on canvas (Art Institute of Chicago)

For the last three decades of his life Renoir devoted himself principally to the nude, which he
considered to be one of the 'indispensable forms' of art. In a succession of studies of seated bathers,
he developed the monumental aspect of the female nude, a far cry from his stylish beauties of the
1870s. *Seated Nude* provides a synthesis of Impressionism and Renoir's own kind of classicism in the
tradition of Rubens.

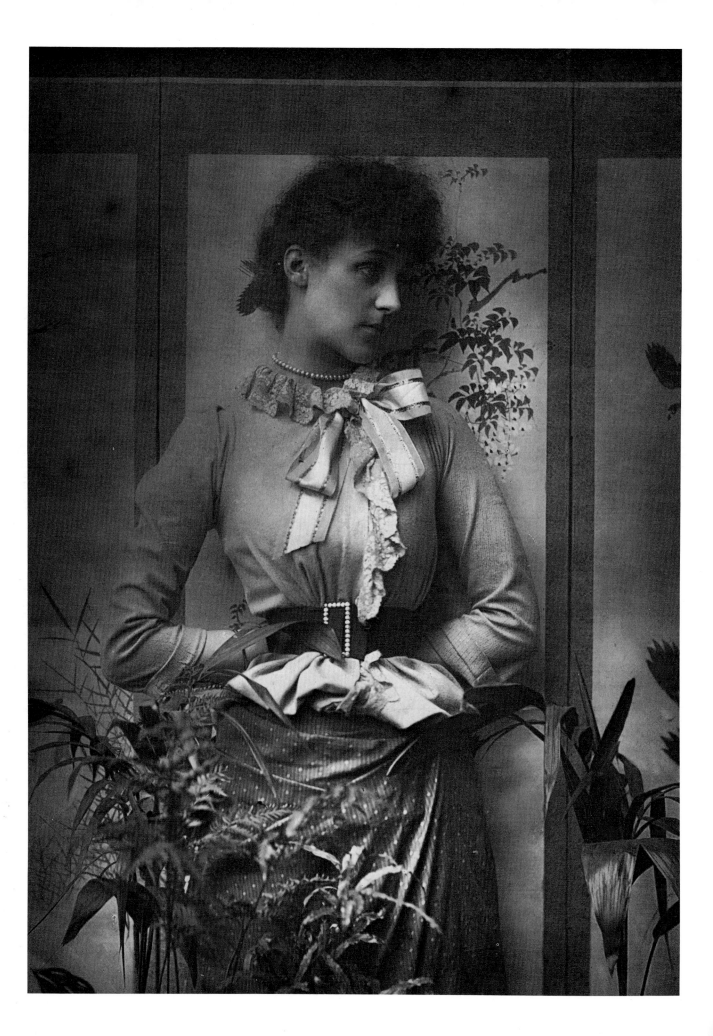

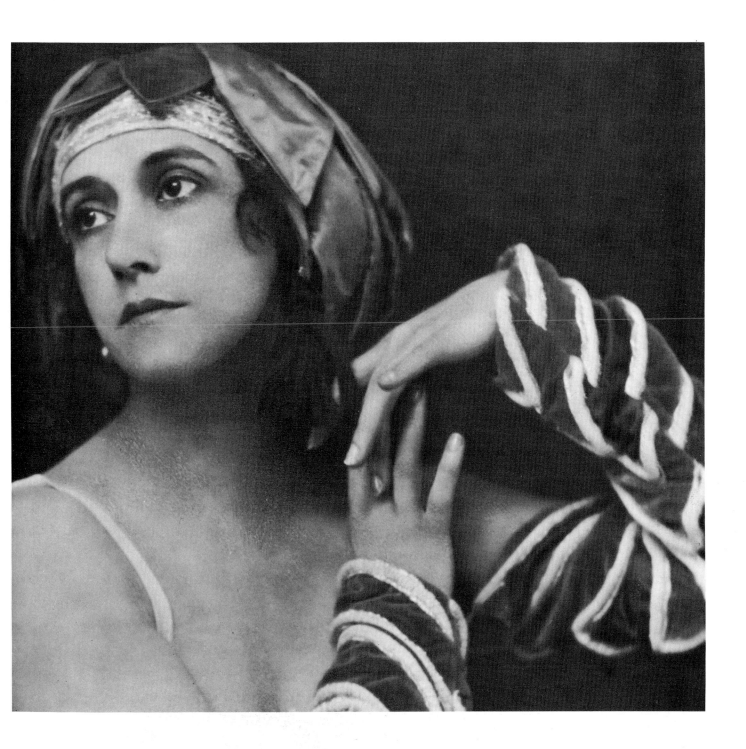

164. OPPOSITE *The Marchioness of Granby*
Photograph (Mansell Collection, London)

The beautiful Marchioness of Granby displays her minute waist and fashionably wistful expression
to perfect advantage in front of a delicate Japanese screen. She was the mother of Lady Diana
Cooper, another celebrated beauty.

165. ABOVE E. O. Hoppé, *Tamara Karsavina*, 1913
Photograph (Mansell Collection, London)

Karsavina came to England with Diaghilev's ballet, of which she was a prima ballerina. Hoppé
photographed many members of the Russian Ballet in his studio, but his portraits of Karsavina,
posing in her costumes for *Carnival* and *Papillons*, were particularly successful.

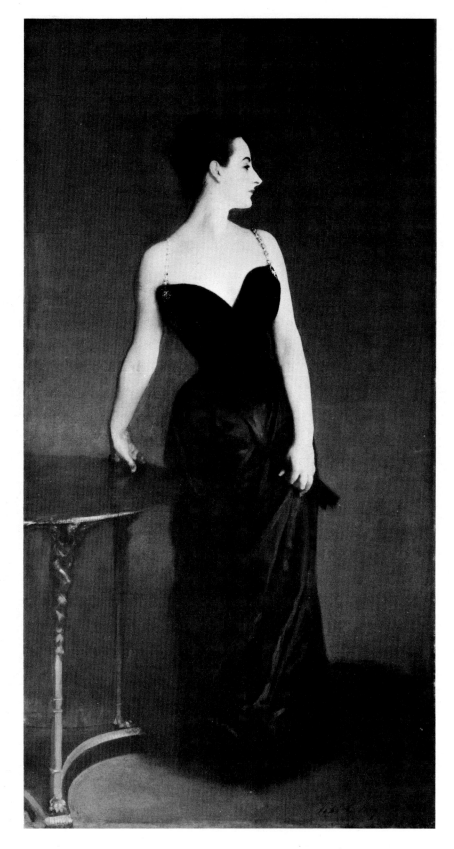

166. John Singer Sargent, *Madame X*, 1884
Oil on canvas (Metropolitan Museum of Art, New York: Arthur H. Hearn Fund, 1916)

Sargent was very attracted to the flashing dark looks of Madame Gautreau, the American-born
wife of a wealthy Parisian banker, and he hoped that his portrait of her would be the greatest
success of the Salon of 1884. It turned out to be his biggest flop, and all Paris mocked her *décolletage*
and the strange lavender tone of her skin. But Sargent maintained that this stark portrait of the
society hostess was the best he had ever done.

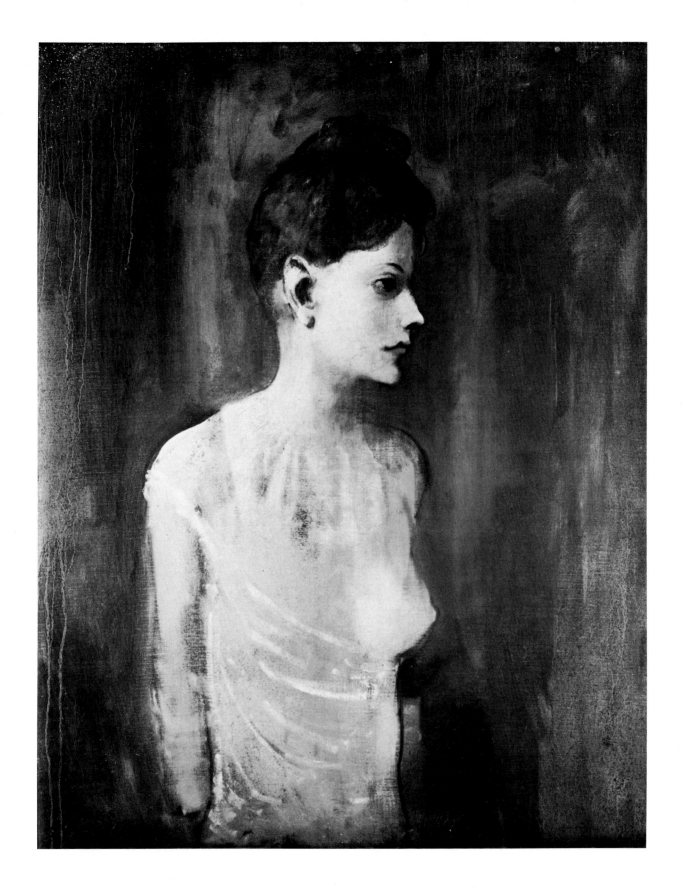

167. Pablo Picasso, *Girl in a Chemise*, 1905
Oil on canvas (Tate Gallery, London)

No painter of comparable status has ever been an stylistically various as Picasso. The paintings of his
Blue Period owe much to the influence of the French artist Puvis de Chavannes who was much
admired in the early 1900s. The dreamy melancholy of 'Blue' paintings such as *Girl in a Chemise*
was soon succeeded by the harsher dynamism of Picasso's early Cubist work.

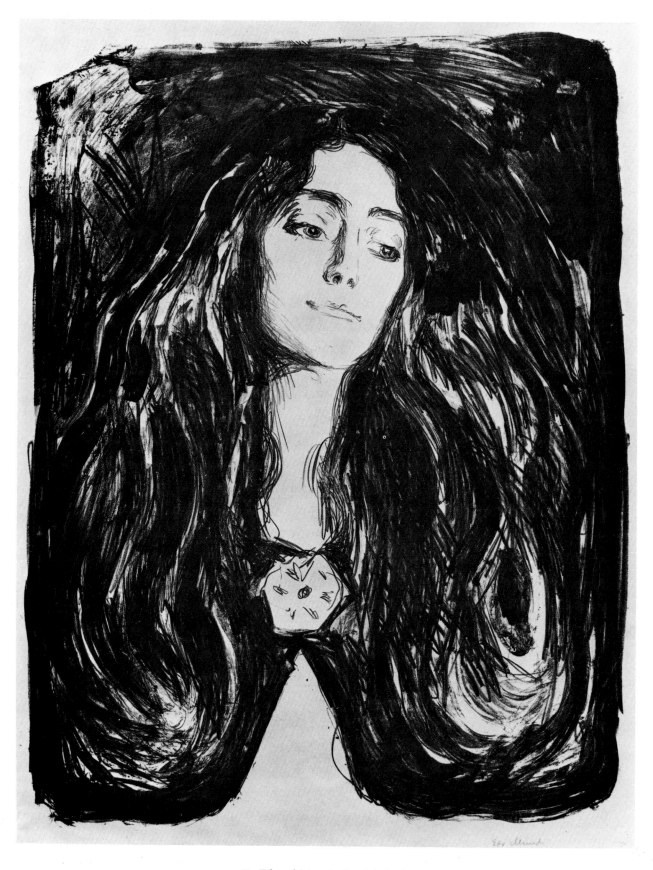

168. Edvard Munch, *Eva Mudocci*, 1903
Lithograph (Brooklyn Museum, New York)

This lyrical portrait of the singer Eva Mudocci, renowned for her beauty as well as her voice, is not
touched with the pathos common to most of Munch's work. The sinuous, waving lines used to
isolate the figure in his famous painting *The Scream* are used here to emphasize Mudocci's luxuriant
hair and to form a magnificent and dramatic frame for her face.

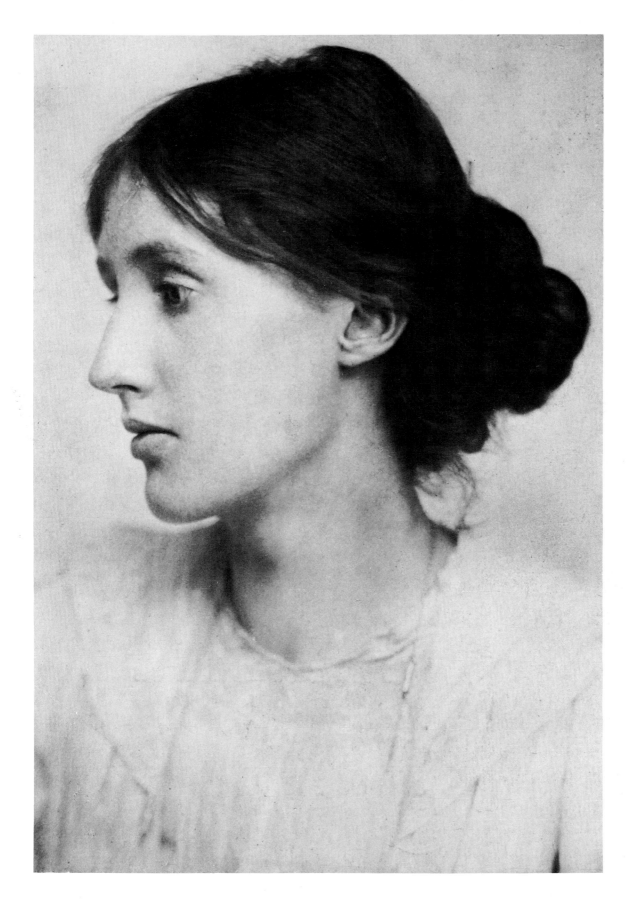

169. J. C. Beresford, *Virginia Woolf*
Photograph (National Portrait Gallery, London)

Virginia Stephens, later the wife of Leonard Woolf, had a highly individual beauty that, although
not classical, perfectly expressed her sensitivity and creative intelligence.

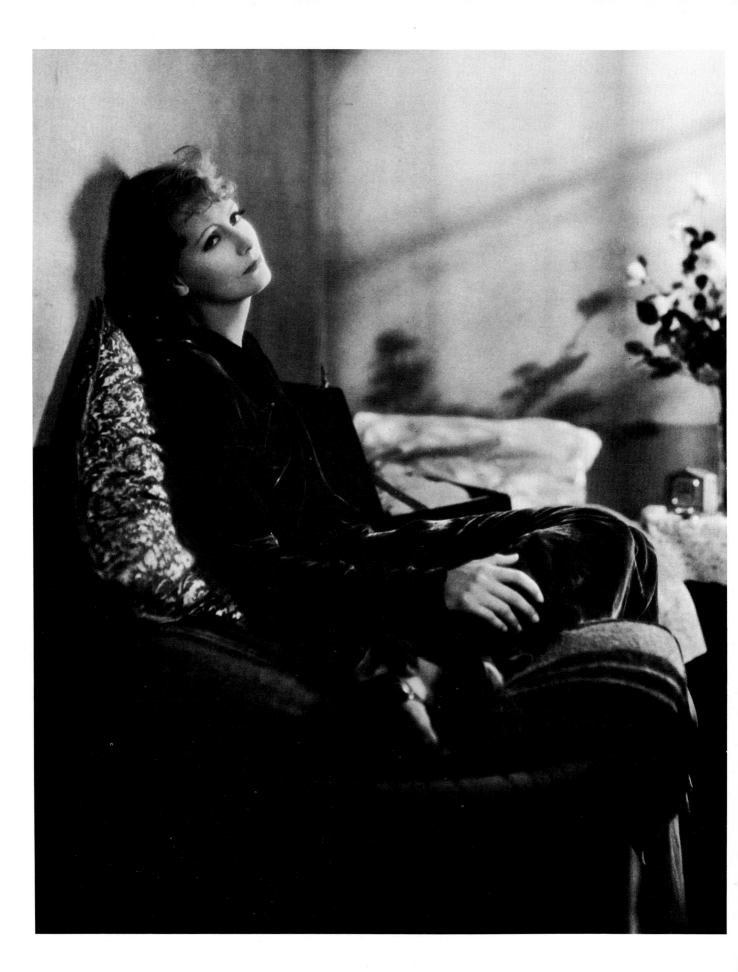

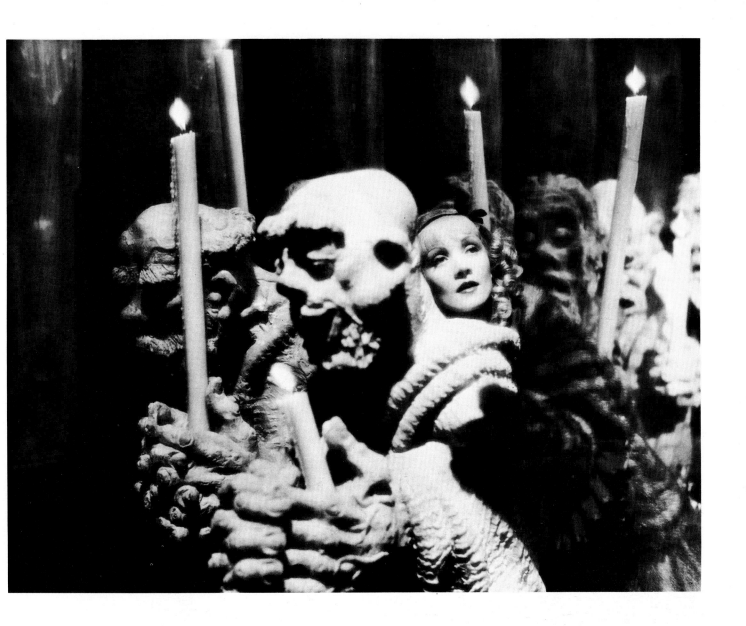

170. OPPOSITE *Greta Garbo*
Still from *The Kiss*, 1929 (MGM)

The timeless and enigmatic nature of Greta Garbo's beauty earned her the name 'The Sphinx', and her austere, melancholy style gave a new emphasis to our conception of the female image. Her languorous pose in this still from *The Kiss* has the controlled eroticism that was part of her fascination.

171. ABOVE *Marlene Dietrich*
Still from *The Scarlet Empress*, 1934 (Paramount Pictures)

Marlene Dietrich combined sophistication with an incandescent glamour, and acquired a legendary mystique in the ominous years before the Second World War. The grotesque figures around her in this scene from *The Scarlet Empress* accentuate her feline delicacy.

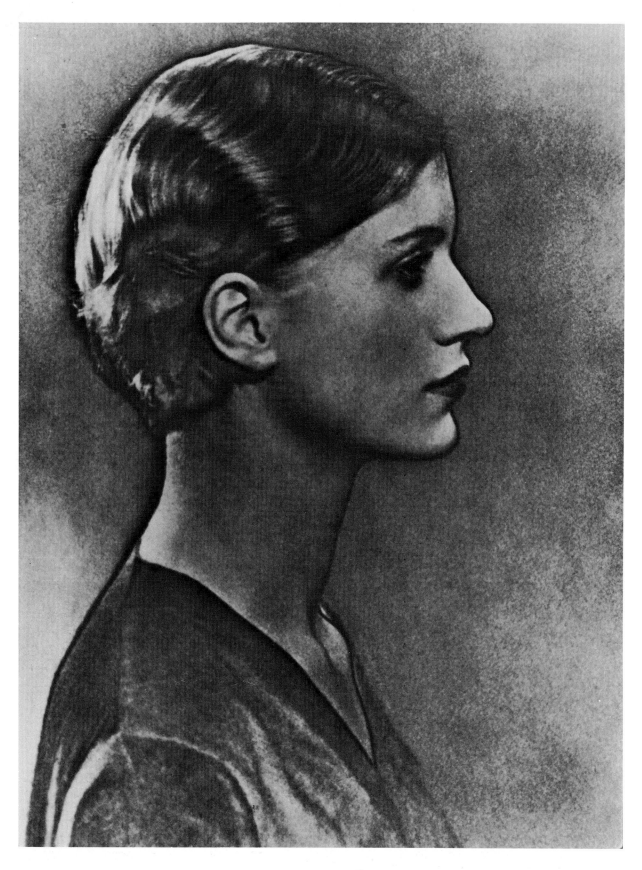

172. Man Ray, *Lee Miller*, *c.* 1932
Solarized photograph (Private Collection)

Man Ray, the Surrealist painter and experimental photographer, made this portrait of his superbly
beautiful model and assistant Lee Miller in the early 1930s. It was then that, quite accidentally, Man
Ray invented the solarized photograph. Solarizing gives a fine dark line round the edge of the
subject and so, as here, sensitively emphasizes the profile.

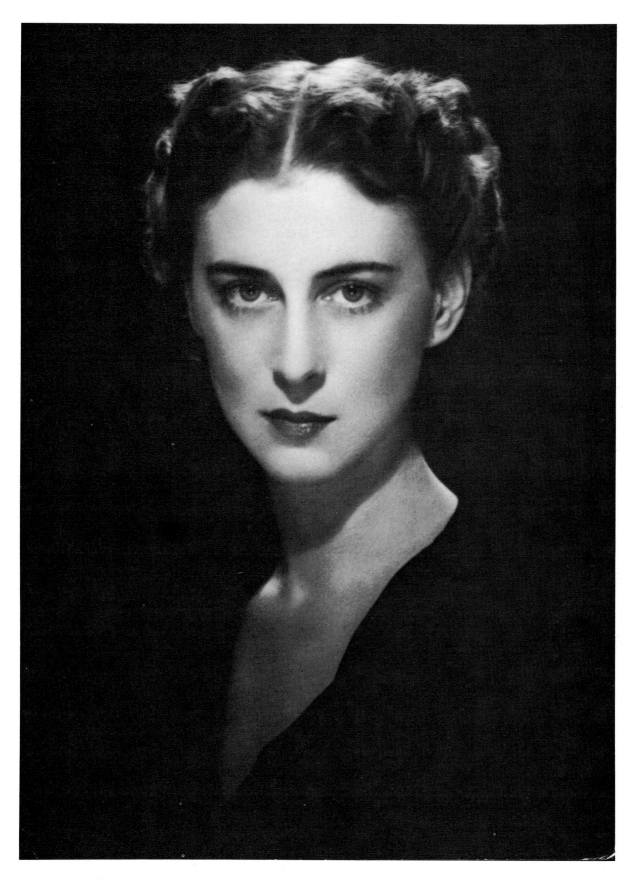

173. Harlipp, *Princess Marina*
Photograph (Weidenfeld and Nicolson Archives, London)

Marina, the youngest daughter of Prince Nicholas of Greece, married the Duke of Kent in the
Autumn of 1934. Her husband was killed in a wartime air crash, but she continued to live in
England, and was much admired for her remarkable beauty and elegance.

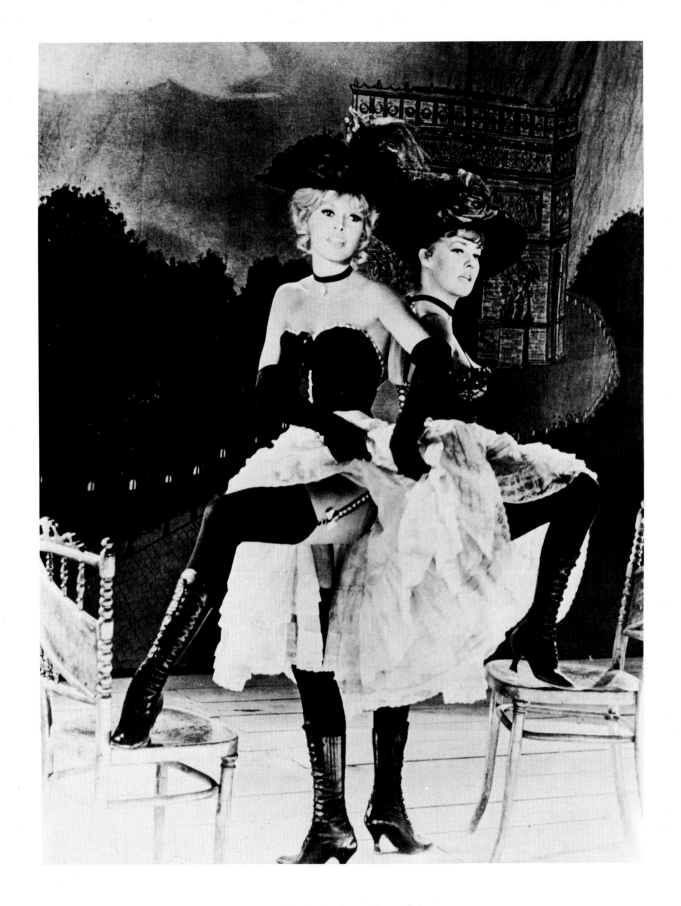

174. *Brigitte Bardot and Jeanne Moreau*
Still from *Viva Maria*, 1965 (United Artists)

In *Viva Maria* the two greatest sex symbols of the 1960s – Brigitte Bardot and Jeanne Moreau –
joined forces in a captivating display that contrasted their very different styles: Bardot innocent but
sexually aggressive and Moreau intelligent, earthy and amoral.

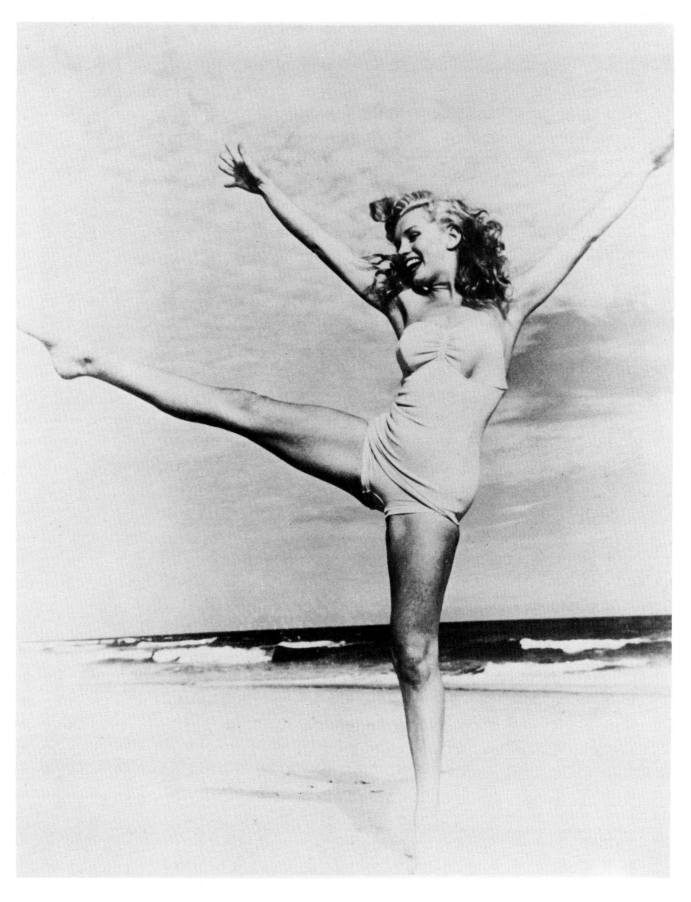

175. *Marilyn Monroe*
Photograph (National Film Archive, London)

The glorious Marilyn Monroe, probably the most famous beauty of our times, doing a high kick
on a beach.

The author and publisher would like to thank the following museums, collections and private individuals by whose kind permission the illustrations are reproduced. Sources without parentheses indicate the owners of paintings and photographs; those within parentheses refer to illustration sources only. The numbers are plate numbers.

1. King Mycerinus between Hathor and the local deity of Diospolis Parva
   Cairo Museum, Egypt (Werner Forman Archive, London)

2. Head of Queen Nefertiti
   Cairo Museum, Egypt (The Mansell Collection, London)

3. Goddess
   Metropolitan Museum of Art, New York

4. Lady Thepu
   Brooklyn Museum, New York: Charles Edwin Wilbour Fund

5. Sky Goddess Nut
   Tanis, Egypt (Weidenfeld and Nicolson Archives, London)

6. Cretan Figurine
   Fitzwilliam Museum, Cambridge

7. Lady with a Wig
   Cairo Museum, Egypt

8. Ludovisi Throne
   Museo Nazionale, Rome

9. Lady of Elche
   Prado, Madrid

10. Peplos Kore
    Acropolis Museum, Athens (Hirmer Fotoarchiv, Munich)

11. Kore
    Acropolis Museum, Athens

12. Kore
    Acropolis Museum, Athens (The Mansell Collection, London)

13. Praxiteles, Head of Aphrodite
    Staatliche Museum, Berlin

14. Mourning Athena
    Acropolis Museum, Athens

15. Demeter of Knidos
    British Museum, London

16. Fury Asleep
    Museo dei Thermes, Rome (Roger-Viollet, Paris)

17. Decadrachm
    Private Collection (Weidenfeld and Nicolson Archives, London)

18. Vase
    National Museum, Athens (Hirmer Fotoarchiv, Munich)

19. Two Tanagrettes
    Louvre, Paris (Giraudon, Paris)

20. Scene from the funeral procession of Ramose (detail)
    Tomb of Ramose, Thebes (Michael Holford Library, Essex)

21. Bust of a Roman Lady
    British Museum, London

22. Head of the Empress Poppea
    Private Collection, London (Weidenfeld and Nicholson Archives, London)

23. Venus de Milo
    Louvre, Paris (Bulloz, Paris)

24. Head of a Goddess
    British Museum, London (Michael Holford Library, Essex)

25. Empress Theodora
    San Vitale, Ravenna (R.B.Fleming, London)

26. Galla Placidia and Her Children
    Brescia Museum

27. Group of women
    Villa Item, Pompeii (Werner Forman Archive, London)

28. French School, Wilton Diptych (right panel)
    National Gallery, London

29. Duccio di Buoninsegna, The Virgin and Child
    (triptych, centre panel)
    National Gallery, London

30. The Virgin of the Visitation (detail)
    Rheims Cathedral (Auguste Allemand, Orsay)

31. Martin Schongauer, Madonna of the Rose Bower
    St Martin's, Colmar (Cooper-Bridgeman Library,
    London)

32. Hans Memlinc, Bathsheba
    Staatsgalerie, Stuttgart

33. Virgin and Child
    Louvre, Paris (Giraudon, Paris)

34. Virgin and Child
    Notre Dame de Grace, Toulouse (Caisse Nationale des
    Monuments Historiques, Paris)

35. Fra Filippo Lippi, The Annunciation
    National Gallery, London

36. Synagoga
    Strasburg Munster (Photo Marburg, Marburg-Lahn)

37. Woman with a Cloak
    Naumburg Cathedral (Helga Schmidt-Glassner,
    Stuttgart)

38. Smiling Woman (detail)
    Naumburg Cathedral (Helga Schmidt-Glassner,
    Stuttgart)

39. Dieric Bouts, Virgin and Child
    Bargello, Florence

40. Dieric Bouts, Entombment (detail)
    National Gallery, London

41. Lucas Cranach the Elder, Cupid Complaining to Venus
    National Gallery, London

42. Ariadne on Naxos
    Bibliothèque Nationale, Paris

43. The Master of Niederrheim, The Charm of Love
    Leipzig Museum

44. Luca della Robbia, Madonna della Mela
    Bargello, Florence (Scala, Florence)

45. Desiderio da Settignano, Virgin and Child
    Philadelphia Museum of Art: The W. P. Wilstach
    Collection

46. Domenico Ghirlandaio, Giovanna Tornabuoni
    Thyssen Collection, Lugano (Foto Brunel, Lugano)

47. Piero di Cosimo, Simonetta Vespucci
    Musée Condé, Chantilly (Lauros-Giraudon, Paris)

48. Piero di Cosimo, A Mythological Subject
    National Gallery, London

49. Leonardo da Vinci, Portrait of a Lady with an Ermine
    (Cecilia Gallerani)
    Czartoryski Museum, Cracow

50. Leonardo da Vinci, Virgin of the Rocks
    Louvre, Paris (Lauros-Giraudon, Paris)

51. Leonardo da Vinci, The Virgin and Child with St Anne
    and St John the Baptist (detail)
    National Gallery, London

52. Leonardo da Vinci, Head of St Anne
    By Gracious Permission of Her Majesty the Queen,
    Windsor Castle Library

53. Leonardo da Vinci, Madonna with the Yard Winder
    Duke of Buccleuch and Queensberry Collection,
    Boughton

54. Piero del Pollaiuolo, Portrait of a Young Woman
    Poldi Pezzoli, Milan (Scala, Florence)

55. Raffaello Sanzio (Raphael), The Three Graces
    Musée Condé, Chantilly (Bulloz, Paris)

56. Raffaello Sanzio (Raphael), La Donna Velata
    Pitti Palace, Florence (Alinari, Florence)

57. Sandro Botticelli, Primavera
    Uffizi, Florence (Scala, Florence)

58. Giorgione, Sleeping Venus (The Dresden Venus)
    Gemaldegalerie, Dresden (Alinari, Florence)

59. Tiziano Vecelli (Titian), Venus of Urbino
    Uffizi, Florence (The Mansell Collection, London)

60. Tiziano Vecelli (Titian), Venus with the Organist
    Prado, Madrid

61. Sandro Botticelli, Birth of Venus (detail)
    Uffizi, Florence (Cooper-Bridgeman Library, London)

62. Raffaello Sanzio (Raphael), Granduca Madonna
    Pitti Palace, Florence (Scala, Florence)

63. Giorgione, Concert Champêtre
    Louvre, Paris (Bulloz, Paris)

64. Tiziano Vecelli (Titian), Sacred and Profane Love
    Borghese Gallery, Rome

65. Tiziano Vecelli (Titian), Venus Anadyomene
    National Gallery of Scotland, Edinburgh

66. Lorenzo Lotto, Triumph of Chastity
    Pallavicini Collection, Rome (Weidenfeld and
    Nicolson Archives, London)

67. Antonio Correggio, The School of Love (Mercury
    instructing Cupid before Venus)
    National Gallery, London

68. Antonio Correggio, Io
    Kunsthistorisches Museum, Vienna

69. Antonio Correggio, Madonna of St Jerome
Pinacoteca, Parma (The Mansell Collection, London)

70. Antonio Correggio, Martyrdom of St Placido and St
Flavia (detail)
Pinacoteca, Parma (The Mansell Collection, London)

71. Agnolo Bronzino, Venus, Cupid, Time and Folly
National Gallery, London

72. Michelangelo Buonarroti, Testa Divina
British Museum, London (Cooper-Bridgeman Library,
London)

73. Michelangelo Buonarroti, Bruges Madonna (detail)
Bruges Cathedral (Ancien Ets Ern, Brussels)

74. Francesco Parmigianino, Madonna del Col Lungo
Uffizi, Florence (Alinari, Florence)

75. Francesco Parmigianino, Antea
Museo Nazionale, Naples.

76. Francesco Parmigianino, Minerva
By Gracious Permission of her Majesty the Queen

77. School of Fontainebleau, Diana of Anet.
Louvre, Paris (Bulloz, Paris)

78. School of Fontainebleau, Diane de Poitiers
Kunstmuseum, Basle

79. Pellegrino Tibaldi, Ulysses Shipwrecked
Palazzo Poggi, Bologna (Weidenfeld and Nicolson
Archives, London)

80. Domenichino, Sibyl
Borghese Gallery, Rome (Alinari, Florence)

81. Annibale Carracci, Madonna and Child with St John
By Gracious Permission of Her Majesty the Queen

82. Giovanni Battista Salvi (Sassoferrato), The Madonna
in Prayer
National Gallery, London

83. Paolo Caliari (Veronese), The Vision of St Helena
National Gallery, London

84. Paolo Caliari (Veronese), Allegory of Vice and Virtue
(detail)
Frick Collection, New York

85. Domenikos Theotocopoulos (El Greco), Virgin and
Child with St Anne
St Vincente Museum, Toledo (Foto Mas, Barcelona)

86. Domenikos Theotocopoulos (El Greco), Lady in a Fur
Wrap
Stirling Maxwell Collection, Pollock House, Glasgow

87. Sir Peter Paul Rubens, The Garden of Love
Prado, Madrid

88. Sir Peter Paul Rubens, The Andromeda
Staatliche Museum, Berlin

89. Sir Peter Paul Rubens, Ildefonso Triptych (centre
panel)
Kunsthistorisches Museum, Vienna

90. Gianlorenzo Bernini, The Blessed Ludovica Albertoni
(detail)
Church of Francesco a Ripa, Rome (The Mansell
Collection, London)

91. Gianlorenzo Bernini, Apollo and Daphne
Borghese Gallery, Rome

92. Paolo Caliari (Veronese), Portrait of a Woman
Louvre, Paris (Giraudon, Paris)

93. Bartolomé Esteban Murillo, The Two Trinities (detail)
National Gallery, London

94. Nicolas Poussin, Sacra Conversazione
National Gallery of Scotland, Edinburgh

95. Guido Reni, Venus and Cupid
Toledo Museum of Art, Ohio

96. Sir Peter Paul Rubens, The Rape of the Sabines
National Gallery, London

97. Rembrandt van Rijn, Hendrickje Stoffels
National Gallery, London

98. Rembrandt van Rijn, Bathsheba
Louvre, Paris

99. Rembrandt van Rijn, Danae
Hermitage, Leningrad (Novosti, London)

100. Rembrandt van Rijn, Lucretia
National Gallery of Art, Washington DC: Andrew W.
Mellon Collection

101. Rembrandt van Rijn, Lucretia
Institute of Arts, Minneapolis (Cooper-Bridgeman
Library, London)

102. Sir Anthony Van Dyck, Queen Henrietta Maria
By Gracious Permission of Her Majesty the Queen

103. Sir Peter Lely, Portrait of a Lady
Aberconway Collection (The Courtauld Institute of
Art, London)

104. Diego Velazquez, The Lady with a Fan
Wallace Collection, London

105. Diego Velazquez, The Toilet of Venus (The Rokeby
Venus)
National Gallery, London

106. Giovanni Battista (Giambattista) Tiepolo, An Allegory
of Venus with Time
National Gallery, London

107. Jean Honoré Fragonard, The Lover Crowned
Frick Collection, New York

108. Antoine Watteau, Fêtes Venetiennes
National Gallery of Scotland, Edinburgh

109. Antoine Watteau, Sheet of Studies
Louvre, Paris (Bulloz, Paris)

110. Thomas Gainsborough, Mary, Countess Howe
The Iveagh Bequest, Kenwood House, London

111. Allan Ramsay, The Painter's Wife
National Gallery of Scotland, Edinburgh

112. Thomas Gainsborough, Mrs Robinson (Perdita)
Wallace Collection, London

113. John Hoppner, Mrs Henry Richmond Gale
Toledo Museum of Art, Ohio: Gift of Edward
Drummond Libbey

114. George Romney, Lady Hamilton as Circe
Tate Gallery, London (John Webb, London)

115. Francisco Goya, Maja Desnuda
Prado, Madrid (Foto Mas, Barcelona)

116. Francisco Goya, Condesa de Chinchon
Duke of Sueca Collection, Madrid (Manso, Madrid)

117. Jean Honoré Fragonard, Young Girl Reading
National Gallery of Art, Washington DC: Jules
S. Bache Collection

118. François Boucher, The Milliner
Nationalmuseum, Stockholm

119. François Boucher, Diana Resting after Her Bath
Louvre, Paris (Cooper-Bridgeman Library, London)

120. François Boucher, The Triumph of Amphitrite
Nationalmuseum, Stockholm

121. François Boucher, Louise O'Murphy
Alte Pinakothek, Munich (The Mansell Collection,
London)

122. Jacques Louis David, Madame Recamier
Louvre, Paris (Cooper-Bridgeman Library, London)

123. Antonio Canova, Paolina Borghese
Borghese Gallery, Rome (Scala, Florence)

124. Jean-Auguste-Dominique Ingres, La Grande Odalisque
Louvre, Paris

125. Jean Baptiste Greuze, Portrait of a Young Girl
Musée de Montepellier (Giraudon, Paris)

126. Jacques Louis David, The Sabine Women
Louvre, Paris (Giraudon, Paris)

127. Théodore Chassériau, Esther
Louvre, Paris (Bulloz, Paris)

128. Jean-Auguste-Dominique Ingres, Comtesse
d'Haussonville
Frick Collection, New York

129. Pierre Paul Prud'hon, The Empress Josephine
Louvre, Paris (Bulloz, Paris)

130. Jean-Auguste-Dominique Ingres, Madame Devauçay
Musée Condé, Chantilly (Bulloz, Paris)

131. Franz Xavier Winterhalter, The Empress Eugénie
Accompanied by her Ladies-in-Waiting
Musée de Compiègne

132. Edouard Manet, Woman with a Parrot
Metropolitan Museum of Art, New York: Gift of
Erwin Davis, 1889

133. Jean-Auguste-Dominique Ingres, La Source
Louvre, Paris (Bulloz, Paris)

134. Jean-Auguste-Dominique Ingres, Le Bain Turc
Louvre, Paris

135. Pierre-Auguste Renoir, Blonde Bather
Sterling and Francine Clark Institute, Williamstown

136. Edouard Manet, Lola de Valence
Louvre, Paris (Bulloz, Paris)

137. Edouard Manet, The Bar at the Folies-Bergères
Courtauld Institute Galleries, London

138. Edouard Manet, Le Déjeuner sur l'Herbe
Jeu de Paume, Paris

139. Edouard Manet, Olympia
Jeu de Paume, Paris

140. Thomas Couture, Odalisque
Cleveland Museum of Art, Ohio

141. Gustave Courbet, Jo, la belle Irlandaise
Nationalmuseum, Stockholm

142. George Frederic Watts, Choosing
National Portrait Gallery, London

143. Richard Buckner, Countess of Cardigan
Private Collection (Weidenfeld and Nicolson Archives,
London)

144. Julia Margaret Cameron, Rosebud Garden of Girls
Royal Photographic Society, London

145. Oscar Gustave Rejlander, Two Women and a Child
The Mansell Collection, London

146. Sir Lawrence Alma-Tadema, In the Tepidarium
Lady Lever Art Gallery, Port Sunlight

147. Sir Edward Burne-Jones, Perseus and his Bride
Southampton Art Gallery

148. Sir Edward Burne-Jones, The Golden Stairs
Tate Gallery, London

149. Sir John Everett Millais, Hearts are Trumps
Tate Gallery, London

150. John Singer Sargent, The Misses Vickers
Sheffield City Art Galleries

151. Albert Moore, Dreamers
Birmingham City Museums and Art Gallery

152. Lord Leighton, Flaming June
Museo de Arte de Ponce, Puerto Rico (Cooper-
Bridgeman Library, London)

153. Dante Gabriel Rossetti, Elizabeth Siddal
Ashmolean Museum, Oxford: F.F.Madan Bequest

154. Jane Morris
Victoria and Albert Museum, London

155. Dante Gabriel Rossetti, The Angel Gabriel Appearing
to the Virgin Mary
Tate Gallery, London

156. Dante Gabriel Rossetti, Beata Beatrix
Tate Gallery, London (John Webb, London)

157. Gaspard Felix Tournachon (Nadar), Sarah Bernhardt
Bibliothèque Nationale, Paris

158. Lily Langtry
The Mansell Collection, London

159. Lily Langtry with Sarah Bernhardt
The Mansell Collection, London

160. Augustus John, Tallulah Bankhead
National Portrait Gallery, Smithsonian Institution,
Washington DC: Gift of the Honourable and Mrs
John Hay Whitney

161. Pierre-Auguste Renoir, La Loge
Courtauld Institute Galleries, London

162. Pierre-Auguste Renoir, Study for The Bathers
Art Institute of Chicago (Bulloz, Paris)

163. Pierre-Auguste Renoir, Seated Nude
Art Institute of Chicago

164. The Marchioness of Granby
The Mansell Collection, London

165. E.O.Hoppé, Tamara Karsavina
The Mansell Collection, London

166. John Singer Sargent, Madame X
Metropolitan Museum of Art, New York: Arthur
H.Hearn Fund, 1916

167. Pablo Picasso, Girl in a Chemise
Tate Gallery, London © S.P.A.D.E.M., Paris, 1980

168. Edvard Munch, Eva Mudocci
Brooklyn Museum, New York

169. J.C.Beresford, Virginia Woolf
National Portrait Gallery, London

170. Greta Garbo
Metro Goldwyn Mayer, Inc., Culver City

171. Marlene Dietrich
Paramount Pictures, New York (National Film
Archive, London)

172. Man Ray, Lee Miller
Private Collection (Weidenfeld and Nicolson Archives,
London) © A.D.A.G.P., Paris, 1980

173. Harlip, Princess Marina
Weidenfeld and Nicolson Archives, London

174. Brigitte Bardot and Jeanne Moreau
United Artists Corporation, New York (National Film
Archive, London)

175. Marilyn Monroe
National Film Archive, London

The publishers have taken all possible care to trace and
acknowledge the ownership of the illustrations. If we have
made an incorrect attribution we apologise and will be
happy to correct the entry in any future reprint, provided
that we receive notification.

AUTHOR'S ACKNOWLEDGMENT

*I would like to thank Miss Julia Brown for
all the help she has given me with this book
at every stage of production.*